Women's Immersion in a Workfare Program: Emerging Challenges for Occupational Therapists

Women's Immersion in a Workfare Program: Emerging Challenges for Occupational Therapists has been co-published simultaneously as *Occupational Therapy in Mental Health*, Volume 23, Numbers 3/4 2007.

Monographic Separates from *Occupational Therapy in Mental Health*™

For additional information on these and other Haworth Press titles, including descriptions, tables of contents, reviews, and prices, use the QuickSearch catalog at http://www.HaworthPress.com.

Women's Immersion in a Workfare Program: Emerging Challenges for Occupational Therapists, by Ellen Greer, PhD (Vol. 23, No 3/4, 2007). *"A MUST NOT ONLY FOR OCCUPATIONAL THERAPISTS, BUT ALSO FOR ALL PRACTITIONERS involved in transitioning people into the workforce, policymakers, and women making this powerful transition." (Pat Precin, MS, OTR/L, Assistant Professor of Occupational Therapy, New York Institute of Technology; Author,* Surviving 9/11: Impact and Experiences of Occupational Therapy Practitioners *and* Healing 9/11: Creative Programming by Occupational Therapists)

Activity Groups in Family-Centered Treatment: Psychiatric Occupational Therapy Approaches for Parents and Children, by Laurette Olson, PhD, OTR/L (Vol. 22, No. 3/4, 2006). *In-depth examination on therapeutic strategies to engage children, adolescents, or parents with mental illness in activities to strengthen parent-child bonds.*

Healing 9/11: Creative Programming by Occupational Therapists, edited by Pat Precin, MS, OTR/L (Vol. 21, No. 3/4, 2006). *"Gives readers valuable insights into the crucial work of skilled helpers– with children, firefighters, psychiatric patients, displaced workers, burn victims, and more–true stories of people helping people cope with and transcend the pain of September 11." (Scott Bennett, MSEd, MSW, Author of* The Elements of Résumé Style)

Occupational Therapy in Forensic Psychiatry: Role Development and Schizophrenia, by Victoria P. Schindler, PhD, OTR (Vol. 20, No. 3/4, 2004). *"DR. SCHINDLER HAS ANSWERED OUR PROFESSION'S CALL for more evidence-based practice by using both basic and applied scientific inquiry to investigate how individuals diagnosed with schizophrenia can develop meaningful life roles while in a maximum-security psychiatric facility. Her findings clearly demonstrate the value of focusing intervention on helping clients pursue meaningful occupations through role development, rather than simply focusing on individual components of treatment." (Laurie Knis-Matthews, OT, MA, Assistant Professor, Kean University)*

Surviving 9/11: Impact and Experiences of Occupational Therapy Practitioners, edited by Pat Precin, MS, OTR/L (Vol. 19, No. 3/4, 2003). *Analyzes the many roles occupational therapy practitioners played during the tragic events of 9/11; examines new therapeutic practices developed because of the terrorist attacks.*

An Ethnographic Study of Mental Health Treatment and Outcomes: Doing What Works, by Fran Babiss, PhD, OTR/L (Vol. 18, No. 3/4, 2002). *"All mental health clinicians and scholars will find this book INSIGHTFUL AND PROVOCATIVE. This book contains more than a description of three women living with anorexia nervosa; the rich qualitative data captures their pain and their struggles with daily life to survive." (Jim Hinojosa, PhD, OT, FAOTA, Professor and Chair, Department of Occupational Therapy, New York University)*

Recovery and Wellness: Models of Hope and Empowerment for People with Mental Illness, edited by Catana Brown, PhD, OTR/L, FAOTA (Vol. 17, No. 3/4, 2001). *Provides guidelines for incorporating wellness and recovery principles into mental health services using the Recovery Model.*

Domestic Abuse Across the Lifespan: The Role of Occupational Therapy, by Christine A. Helfrich, PhD, OTR/L (Vol. 16, No. 3/4, 2001). *"For those occupational therapists who view themselves as holistic service providers, this book is a must-read. . . . Includes examples, studies, and research results." (Linda T. Learneard, OTR/L, President, Occupational Therapy Consultation and Rehabilitation Services, Inc.)*

Brain Injury and Gender Role Strain: Rebuilding Adult Lifestyles After Injury, by Sharon A. Gutman, PhD, OTR (Vol. 15, No. 3/4, 2000). *"Dr. Gutman has developed an innovative target setting and treatment planning protocol that focuses the therapist on the key areas of concern.*

I highly recommend this book to therapists who work with clients in the post-acute period of recovery from TBI." (Gordon Muir Giles, MA, Dip COT, OTR, Director of Neurobehavioral Services, Crestwood Behavioral Health, Inc., and Assistant Professor, Samuel Merritt College, Oakland, California)

New Frontiers in Psychosocial Occupational Therapy, edited by Anne Hiller Scott, PhD, OTR, FAOTA (Vol. 14, No. 1/2, 1998). *"Speaks a clear message about mental health practice in occupational therapy, shattering old visions of practice to insights about empowerment and advocacy."* (Sharan L. Schwartzberg, EdD, OTR, FAOTA, Professor and Chair, Boston School of Occupational Therapy, Tufts University)

Evaluation and Treatment of the Psychogeriatric Patient, edited by Diane Gibson, MS, OTR (Vol. 10, No. 3, 1991). *"Occupational therapists everywhere, learners and sophisticates alike, and in-hospital and out-patient areas as well as home-bound and home-active, would enjoy and profit from this exposition as much as I did."* (American Association of Psychiatric Administrators)

Student Recruitment in Psychosocial Occupational Therapy: Intergenerational Approaches, edited by Susan Haiman (Vol. 10, No. 1, 1990). *"Can serve to enlighten both academics and clinicians as to their roles in attracting students to become practitioners in mental health settings. Each article could well serve as a catalyst for discussion in the classroom or clinic."* (Canadian Journal of Occupational Therapy)

Group Protocols: A Psychosocial Compendium, edited by Susan Haiman (Vol. 9, No. 4, 1990). *"Presents succinct protocols for a wide range of groups that are typically run by activities therapists, vocational counselors, art therapists, and other mental health professionals."* (International Journal of Group Psychotherapy)

Instrument Development in Occupational Therapy, edited by Janet Hawkins Watts and Chestina Brollier (Vol. 8, No. 4, 1989). *Examines content and concurrent validity and development of the Assessment of Occupational Functioning (AOF), and carefully compares the AOF with a similar instrument, the Occupational Case Analysis Interview and Rating Scale (OCAIRS), to discover the similarities and strengths of these instruments.*

Group Process and Structure in Psychosocial Occupational Therapy, edited by Diane Gibson, MS, OTR (Vol. 8, No. 3, 1989). *Highly skilled professionals examine the important concepts of group therapy to help build cohesive, safe groups.*

Treatment of Substance Abuse: Psychosocial Occupational Therapy Approaches, edited by Diane Gibson, MS, OTR (Vol. 8, No. 2, 1989). *A unique overview of contemporary assessment and rehabilitation of alcohol and chemical dependent substance abusers.*

The Development of Standardized Clinical Evaluations in Mental Health, Principal Investigator: Noomi Katz, PhD, OTR; edited by Claudia Kay Allen, MA, OTR, FAOTA; Commentator: Janice P. Burke, MA, OTR, FAOTA (Vol. 8, No. 1, 1988). *"Contains a collection of research-based articles encompassing several evaluations that can be used by occupational therapists practicing in mental health."* (American Journal of Occupational Therapy)

Evaluation and Treatment of Adolescents and Children, edited by Diane Gibson, MS, OTR (Vol. 7, No. 2, 1987). *Experts share research results and practices that have proven successful in helping young people who suffer from psychiatric and medical disorders.*

Treatment of the Chronic Schizophrenic Patient, edited by Diane Gibson, MS, OTR (Vol. 6, No. 2, 1986). *"Reflect[s] creative and fresh concepts of current treatment for the chronically mentally ill. . . . Recommended for the therapist practicing in psychiatry."* (Canadian Journal of Occupational Therapy)

The Evaluation and Treatment of Eating Disorders, edited by Diane Gibson, MS, OTR (Vol. 6, No. 1, 1986). *"A wealth of information. . . . Covers the subject thoroughly. . . . This book, well-conceived and well-written, is recommended not only for clinicians working with clients with anorexia nervosa and bulimia but for all therapists who wish to become acquainted with the subject of eating disorders in general."* (Library Journal)

Philosophical and Historical Roots of Occupational Therapy, edited by Karen Diasio Serrett (Vol. 5, No. 3, 1985). *"Recommended as an easy-to-get-through background read for occupational therapists and for generalists wishing a fuller acquaintance with the backdrop of occupational therapy."* (Rehabilitation Literature)

Women's Immersion in a Workfare Program: Emerging Challenges for Occupational Therapists

Ellen Greer, PhD

Women's Immersion in a Workfare Program: Emerging Challenges for Occupational Therapists has been co-published simultaneously as *Occupational Therapy in Mental Health*, Volume 23, Numbers 3/4 2007.

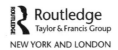

Routledge
Taylor & Francis Group

NEW YORK AND LONDON

First Published by

The Haworth Press, Inc., 10 Alice Street, Binghamton, NY 13904-1580

Published by Routledge
711 Third Avenue, New York, NY 10017
2 Park Square, Milton Park, Abingdon, Oxon, OX14 4RN

Women's Immersion in a Workfare Program: Emerging Challenges for Occupational Therapists has been co-published simultaneously as *Occupational Therapy in Mental Health*™, Volume 23, Numbers 3/4 2007.

Library of Congress Cataloging-in-Publication Data

Greer, Ellen.
    Women's immersion in a workfare program : emerging challenges for occupational therapists / Ellen Greer.
        p. cm.
    "Women's immersion in a workfare program : emerging challenges for occupational therapists has been co-published simultaneously as Occupational therapy in mental health, volume 23, Numbers 3/4 2007."
    Includes bibliographical references and index.
    ISBN 978-0-7890-3028-3 (hard cover : alk. paper) – ISBN 978-0-7890-3029-0 (soft cover : alk. paper)
        1. Temporary Assistance for Needy Families (Program) 2. Welfare recipients–Employment–United States–Case studies. 3. Occupational training for women–United States–Case studies. I. Occupational therapy in mental health II. Title.
    HV95.G695 2007
    362.83'84–dc22
                                                                                                2008000090

Publisher's Note
The publisher has gone to great lengths to ensure the quality of this reprint but points out that some imperfections in the original may be apparent.

Women's Immersion
in a Workfare Program:
Emerging Challenges
for Occupational Therapists

CONTENTS

ABOUT THE AUTHOR

Ellen Greer, PhD, OTR/L, is Assistant Professor in the Department of Occupational Therapy at the New York Institute of Technology. She has been an occupational therapist for over 30 years and is also trained and licensed in psychoanalysis. Her research interests focus on the transitions women confront in health, education, work and family life.

Recently becoming a grandmother, Dr. Greer cherishes the continuity of life and the expressions of courage, strength and love that bind a family through the generations.

Acknowledgments

I have been blessed to have encountered extraordinary individuals on my path to completing this dissertation. With gratitude, I thank my Committee–Dr. Deborah R. Labovitz, Chairperson; Dr. Margot Ely; and Dr. Judy Grossman.

Their wisdom, guidance, unwavering support, and invaluable feedback during every stage of the dissertation process helped me to grow. Their influence as role models and mentors has been immeasurable.

I will always be thankful to Dr. Jim Hinojosa for his help and clarity along the way, and to Dr. Mary V. Donohue who has mentored me with great generosity throughout the years. I thank Marie-Louise Blount, along with Jim and Mary for giving me scholarly opportunities.

With admiration, I thank Dr. Anne Cronin Mosey for the precious time I spent learning in her classes.

I wish to thank Dr. Sandee McClowery for providing a formative learning experience in the first year of my doctoral studies. Both she and Pamela Gailhouse influenced the direction of my research.

I thank Carol Capello for her sensitive understanding of the dissertation process and her remarkable editorial assistance.

Without the support of the nursing home administration and staff this dissertation would not have been possible. It is with much appreciation that I thank them and the courageous participants of the study–Agnes, Betty, Connie, Dolores, Esther, and Florence.

When I think of the layers of preparation needed to complete a dissertation both emotionally and intellectually I must thank all of my teachers, supervisors, fellow students and colleagues that have touched my life throughout my psychoanalytic training and doctoral studies.

[Haworth co-indexing entry note]: "Acknowledgments." Greer, Ellen. Co-published simultaneously in *Occupational Therapy in Mental Health* (The Haworth Press, Inc.) Vol. 23, No. 3/4, 2007, pp. xix-xx; and: *Women's Immersion in a Workfare Program: Emerging Challenges for Occupational Therapists* (Ellen Greer) The Haworth Press, Inc., 2007, pp. xv-xvi. Single or multiple copies of this article are available for a fee from The Haworth Document Delivery Service [1-800-HAWORTH, 9:00 a.m. - 5:00 p.m. (EST). E-mail address: docdelivery@haworthpress.com].

xv

I had the good fortune to have colleagues who listened to my research ideas, read chapter drafts, and offered friendship that will always be remembered. Veronica Golos, Sharon Gutman, Charles Ippolito, Michelle Mills, Marianne Mortera, Marjorie Sczcepanski, Anne H. Scott, Sheri Wadler, and Suzanne White–I thank you. To my early support group– Vicki Irang, Tai McConnell, and Awilda Ramos–I offer my appreciation for the time we worked together.

For their inspiration during the time of working on the dissertation, I thank my support group–Lauren, Liz, Judy, Isabel, Mayo, Toby, Gillian, Lucinda, John and Laurie–and my Qi Gong classmates. Throughout the dissertation process, I had the pleasure of talking with a group of individuals who provided me with emotional support under the most trying of times. I thank Steve Borton, Ernest Brod, Sherry Ceridan, Ira Jacobs, Carol Lerner, Rose and Paul McAloon, Lucy Paccione, Patricia Panella, Gene Smithberg, and Alma Weisberg.

For their dedication, talent, and support in helping me toward facilitating the healing process, I thank with all my heart Dr. Jei Atacama, Dr. Aviva Atacama, Debbie Atacama, Evelyn Aguayo, Dr. Mingxia Li, and Dr. Nan Lu.

I give my deepest appreciation to Dr. George Raptis for his healing nature and for being there to help me with his knowledge at the most critical moment, as well as to Dr. Martin S. Goldstein and Dr. Sharon Diamond for their excellent care. I also thank Rita Gurrey, RN, for her healing sense of humor.

My heartfelt gratitude goes to Dr. Theodore Laquercia for being a fine teacher and training analyst.

My mother, Pearl Haber, my uncle and aunt, Heli H. Miller and Mildred Ockey, my sisters, Lorraine Fried and Diane Haber, cousins Fred Mendelsohn, Maressa and Marc Gershowitz and friends Amy Moulton, Jean Osnos, Toby Kaplowitz and Geraldine Herrin have been dear to me through many difficult and happy hours in my life. Thank you.

With my love and affection, I thank my husband Edward for his dearest devotion to me always, and to our family, Brian, Stefanie and infant Charlotte Rose and Daniel and Francine, who enrich our lives with joy and happiness.

I dedicate this dissertation to my family members who are no longer here but who live in my heart: my father, George Haber; my grandparents, Phillip and Rose Miller; my aunt, Charlotte Mendelsohn and granddaughter Olivia Hope Greer.

Preface

It has been over a decade since President Clinton signed the Personal Responsibility and Work Opportunity Act of 1996 that replaced the traditional welfare system, Aid to Families with Dependent Children (AFDC), with Temporary Assistance for Needy Families (TANF). Welfare reform now required work or preparation for work as a condition for receiving benefits. Hailed as a great success, the workfare program did help many families become self-sufficient, but on closer examination, the most vulnerable families did not succeed. Policy analysts began to focus on low income families with children and the significant barriers to employment, child and family well-being. The next step was to understand the diversity of outcomes and the complexity of issues associated with success.

To understand the nuances it is necessary to examine welfare reform on an individual level–through personal narratives. This book describes the stories of six women who cycled through the workfare program but did not make the transition to sustained employment. Their stories illustrate the barriers that affect work and family life as well as the factors that explain resilience in face of significant hardship. The women's lives are described in rich detail so that we feel their struggle and come to understand that they have *promises to keep*.

Dolores, Betty, Florence, Agnes, Connie and Esther were all assigned to an occupational therapy clinic in a nursing home for their workfare placement. They each experience multiple risk factors from their past and current living situations, including family disruption, mental illness, homelessness, addiction and incarceration, health problems, abuse and domestic violence.[1] At least one child in each family had serious problems such as physical or mental illness, behavioral problems and/or school failure. The competing demands of work and parenting created *role distress* and difficulty performing the multiple tasks that are part of

[Haworth co-indexing entry note]: "Preface." Grossman, Judy. Co-published simultaneously in *Occupational Therapy in Mental Health* (The Haworth Press, Inc.) Vol. 23, No. 3/4, 2007, pp. xxi-xxii; and: *Women's Immersion in a Workfare Program: Emerging Challenges for Occupational Therapists* (Ellen Greer) The Haworth Press, Inc., 2007, pp. xvii-xviii. Single or multiple copies of this article are available for a fee from The Haworth Document Delivery Service [1-800-HAWORTH, 9:00 a.m. - 5:00 p.m. (EST). E-mail address: docdelivery@haworthpress.com].

xvii

motherwork. Worry and caretaking responsibilities spilled over into the workplace.

What makes the women remarkable, however, is their resilience and ability to survive adversity. It is not their lack of desire but the lack of support that led to insecurity and continued unemployment.

The findings from this study are consistent with the cumulative evidence from welfare research.[2] Without adequate supports–educational opportunities, childcare and financial incentives–there will be limited success and children will suffer. In particular, the impact on adolescent school performance is troubling. The lesson learned from retrospective studies is that severely disadvantaged women made the least gains, suggesting that the intergenerational cycle of poverty and associated risk factors will continue.

The women's voices should give shape to policy and we need to heed their recommendations. Education, literacy skills and professional development are necessary to move families towards economic security rather than simply prepare them for low-wage employment. Working mothers have multiple roles and responsibilities, not just to increase family income but to raise healthy and socially responsible children who can become self-sufficient as they reach adulthood.

This book offers some universal themes–the struggle to manage work and family life, and the resilience of the human mind and spirit to overcome adversity and create a better life for one's children. The women you will meet in this book share these universal themes without the supports and opportunities to overcome the barriers that impede success. The narrow focus on employment limited our ability to help the most vulnerable welfare mothers and their children. There is no quick fix. The risk factors for unemployment are similar to the risk factors for inadequate parenting and child well-being. Through qualitative methods, this study reached the same conclusions that policymakers now endorse, to dedicate adequate resources to help women fulfill both work and parenting responsibilities.

Judy Grossman

REFERENCES

1. Knitzer, J. (2000). Promoting resilience: Helping young children and parents affected by substance abuse, domestic violence, and depression in the context of welfare reform. New York: The National Center for Children in Poverty.

2. Cauthen, N.K. (2006). Looking forward, looking back. Reflections on the 10th anniversary of welfare reform. New York: National Center for Children in Poverty.

Chapter 1

Introduction

*The mark of a noble society is to be found, not in the manner in
which it helps the rich, but in how it helps the poor. Not in its vir-
tues during good times, but in its character during hard times. Not
in how it protects the powerful, but in how it defends the vulnerable. These are the attributes by which a great society should be
judged.* (Rank, 1994, p. 204)

Over five million families, mostly headed by single women receiving
Temporary Assistance for Needy Families (TANF), have been caught in
the current changes in welfare reform. For 60 years, welfare benefits had
been available to eligible families, with minimal expectations to meet
work requirements and no time limit to achieve self-sufficiency (Mink,
1998). However, all that changed when President Clinton signed into law
the Personal Responsibility and Work Opportunity Reconciliation Act
(PRA) on August 26, 1996. The long-term entitlement Aid to Families
with Dependent Children (AFDC) was abolished and replaced with TANF,
a five-year time-limited benefit program requiring participation in work
activities (Keen, 1997; Wittman, 1998).

The purpose behind the new TANF program is to provide assistance to
needy families with or expecting children, and to provide parents with job
preparation, work and support services to enable them to leave the program and become self-sufficient (Mink & Solinger, 2003). The new legislation authorizes the government to provide states with block grants so
that they can implement welfare reform within a general set of guidelines.
In a trend towards devolution, the government has authorized states to

[Haworth co-indexing entry note]: "Introduction." Greer, Ellen. Co-published simultaneously in
Occupational Therapy in Mental Health (The Haworth Press, Inc.) Vol. 23, No. 3/4, 2007, pp. 1-6; and:
Women's Immersion in a Workfare Program: Emerging Challenges for Occupational Therapists (Ellen
Greer) The Haworth Press, 2007, pp. 1-6. Single or multiple copies of this article are available for a fee from The
Haworth Document Delivery Service [1-800-HAWORTH, 9:00 a.m. - 5:00 p.m. (EST). E-mail address:
docdelivery@haworthpress.com].

Available online at http://otmh.haworthpress.com
© 2007 by The Haworth Press, Inc. All rights reserved.
doi:10.1300/J004v23n03_01

move large numbers of welfare recipients into the workforce through a workfare process (Koon, 1997). Workfare, a concept that emerged from Nixon's *New Federalism* of 1969, has emerged as a social contract requiring obligatory work in exchange for a time-limited welfare benefit (Koon, 1997; Nathan, 1993). Today, workfare aims to move TANF recipients, both men and women, off the welfare rolls to employment over a five year period while earning their benefit through participating in work-related activities. In 1996, almost 80% of the TANF population were single mothers with children (O'Hara, 2002). At that time, 17.5% of all households were headed by females without a spouse, while only 4.4% were headed by males without a spouse (Robles, 1997). Clearly, welfare reform would have a major impact on the lives of the more than 200,000 single women with children in New York City who were TANF recipients, given the demands of motherhood and heading a household.

Single mothers with children have a complex transition to make in light of this recent legislation (Blank & Blum, 1997). The road to becoming self-sufficient through the mandatory work program impacts their roles as mothers and providers and ultimately affects the future of their children (Smith, 1995; Zaslow & Emig, 1997). Researchers examining the relationship between low-income mothers going to work and the effects on their children have rarely explored the natural transitional experience of mothers moving into workfare, including the multiple role challenges that lie ahead of them as mothers engaged in moving towards self-sufficiency (Kisker & Ross, 1997; Parcel & Menaghan, 1997). Currently, it is the women in workfare who are usually caring for the children and have to cope with complex issues and problems. Describing what occurs in this natural transition by studying women's experiences might lend insight into the nature of the challenges these women face in workfare, as well as the strategies they choose to resolve their problems.

In a resource manual that helps prepare women make the transition from welfare to work through education, Lepak, Stokes, and Harder (1994-1995) explain that barriers such as fear, guilt, and low self-esteem have prevented welfare-reliant women with children from making educational and work transitions in their lives. Brong (1996) points out other significant barriers to employment, such as inadequate social supports, lack of job skills, domestic violence, physical/mental disabilities, histories of substance abuse and addiction, and long-term welfare dependency. These obstacles cut across race and ethnicity and are often experienced by single-parent Workfare participants in both rural and inner-city locales (Brong, 1996; Delsman, WNYC, 1997; Perlmutter, 1997; Rank, 1994).

WORKFARE PROGRAM

How does a workfare program respond to female TANF recipients? How are individual needs of female participants in workfare assessed? How are training and support services tailored to help them in this transition? These questions address a scope of community practice in the field of occupational therapy developed to enable individuals to make the transition to work.

I became interested in these questions when I came into contact with women workfare participants assigned to work at an occupational therapy clinic in a nursing home where I had worked. I had the opportunity to talk with them and to listen to their views about and experiences with the program, as well as how they felt about and how they managed being workfare participants and mothers. I began to notice that some women moved through the program more smoothly than others and that some even dropped out. I wanted to understand more about their experiences from their perspective so that I could learn how to best work together. I found no related documentation in the research literature.

AVA AND SONNY

The stories of Ava and Sonny whom I met at the occupational therapy clinic at the nursing home describe the interweaving of two mothers' resilient effort to make the transition to workfare participant and some particular barriers to employment. Single mothers of young children and TANF recipients, Ava and Sonny had been notified of their mandated workfare assignment in the winter of 1996. Financial and medical needs made both women decide to maintain the TANF benefit. They began to adjust to finding adequate child and health care so that they could start the mandated workfare program. The program, consisting of a sequence of four modules (basic education/work experience, job club, work experience, job club) over a one-year period, can be repeated for up to five years if employment is not obtained.

Ava, a single mother of two young children, a recovering drug addict, and a high school dropout, was coping with the complexities of obtaining early intervention services for her one-year-old daughter diagnosed with cerebral palsy.

She often felt overwhelmed and anxious dealing with her own recovery process. These difficult feelings, along with caring for a special needs infant and demanding toddler, created an intense life experience. Whenever possible, Ava worked off the books to manage her expenses.

Sonny, a single mother, had been focusing her energies on her school-age son who has a hearing impairment and requires ongoing medical care with intermittent surgeries. She hoped that entering the workfare program would provide an opportunity for her to obtain some job skills. Sonny had a history of unsuccessful job experiences, usually because of interpersonal difficulties that erupted in her work relationships. Her previous work experiences had left her feeling hopeless and with low self-confidence.

Up until this time, both women had been welfare reliant for several years, using their benefit for rent and food. Ava and Sonny had found they could not make it on welfare benefits alone and had developed strategies to survive. C. Turner (1997) calls this ability to form strategies a "learned talent to survive" (p. 162). These strategies included doing "off-the-books" jobs, such as babysitting, cleaning apartments, or caring for an elderly neighbor. With the new workfare requirement, they had to give up these activities to be present at the workfare setting. Both women found that not being able to earn additional needed income placed them in a critical situation. They also realized that with a five-year time limit to the TANF benefit, their safety net for survival would disappear unless they could earn a competitive wage (Edin & Lein, 1997). Both women realized that without an education they were targeted for occupationally segregated jobs, such as domestic work or nurse's aid assignments (Higgenbotham & Romero, 1997).

The year that I met Ava and Sonny, they were already familiar with the workfare program which they and other participants across the country term the circle (K. Rhoades, Coordinator, Women in Transition Program, University of Wisconsin-Eau Claire (personal communication, January, 1997)). "The circle" is considered repetitively passing through the program as a result of not obtaining employment (personal communication with anonymous workfare participant, May 1997).

Ava found the work in the occupational therapy clinic interesting and had a gift for connecting with the most withdrawn residents. However, external factors began to interfere with her progress in the clinic. Without social supports to help with childcare in the mornings and pediatric clinic appointments, she would frequently arrive late or be absent. When the staff spoke with her about this, she revealed that her experience moving into a new role as a workfare participant was stressful and exasperating. She knew of other women in similar circumstances who wanted to kill themselves. This dire reaction to a forced work transition has been reported by workfare participants in other settings (Dr. Harrigan, Director of Cope Program, Laguardia Community College, personal communication, October 1998; Mink, 1998). Ava experienced stress when taking on new roles and responsibilities, eventually developed an illness, and then began to miss consecutive days at the clinic. In time, she dropped out of the workfare program, and no one knew what subsequently happened to her. In contrast, Sonny initially disliked the clinic setting and felt inadequate to help the frail older nursing home residents. Slowly, she reported feeling tenderness toward the residents, and her attitude and appearance revealed her increased self-confidence. She asked for more responsibility each day, and she seemed to enjoy the clerical activities that took her to different parts of the nursing home. Concerned that she had often lost jobs quickly, she viewed the workfare experience as a chance to pay attention to her work problems. The last I heard about Sonny, she was still continuing in the program.

These are just two stories. But not enough is known about women's individual cultural experiences as they move from the role of welfare recipient to that of workfare volunteer. How do they find meaning in their experiences of forced transition? Do they view the experience as a loss of choice, not being able to stay home with their children, or as a window of opportunity to confront difficulties to resolve resistances to personal barriers to employment? The literature rarely represents the perspectives of TANF women's experiences in workfare, in contrast to the outspoken voices of media and political debate. The activities, interactions, and relationships that may be linked to what constitutes success or failure in the transition to work have not been fully described by TANF women participants themselves.

DIRECT NARRATIVES

V.W. Turner (1986) discusses how meaning emerges from experience, how meaning occurs through merging the synthesis of culture and language from the past with our wishes, thoughts and feelings in the present. In any rehabilitation process, change is a series of gains and setbacks, and what may feel like failure can be a step towards accomplishment (Kreuger, 1984). Thus, it is important to gather information from the narratives directly from TANF women. As Jencks (1997) notes, programs for single mothers in this country will only be improved if legislators know the effects of TANF on these women's lives. This proposed study provides such insights.

In this study, I describe, analyze, and interpret the narratives of six women to understand their reported experiences of workfare as preparation for employment. I identify patterns and themes that emerge in their narratives in order to address the following research questions:

1. How do these women receiving TANF experience the mandatory work program as preparation for transition into the workforce?
2. How do the women fit this mandatory program into their daily life?
3. How do these women feel about this transition into the workforce?

doi:10.1300/J004v23n03_01

Chapter 2

Single Mothers' Transition
to Self-Sufficiency

SUMMARY. In this chapter, I review the literature in four sections central to my research questions. First, I review the socio-historical context of
trends that have had an impact on single mothers in transition from economic assistance to self-sufficiency. Next, I present research that focuses
on poor women's interactions with barriers to work versus self-sufficiency. Then I examine the reported interactions between work, family
role strain, and the psychological well-being of low-income women
during their transition to work. Finally, I introduce related literature
that reflects studies and reports on the outcomes of TANF after 1996.
doi:10.1300/J004v23n03_02 *[Article copies available for a fee from The Haworth
Document Delivery Service: 1-800-HAWORTH. E-mail address: <docdelivery@
haworthpress.com> Website: <http://www.HaworthPress.com> © 2007 by The
Haworth Press, Inc. All rights reserved.]*

KEYWORDS. Role strain, barriers to self-sufficiency, kinship systems,
well-being, mental health

[Haworth co-indexing entry note]: "Single Mothers' Transition to Self-Sufficiency." Greer, Ellen.
Co-published simultaneously in *Occupational Therapy in Mental Health* (The Haworth Press, Inc.) Vol. 23,
No. 3/4, 2007, pp. 7-23; and: *Women's Immersion in a Workfare Program: Emerging Challenges for Occupa-
tional Therapists* (Ellen Greer) The Haworth Press, 2007. pp. 7-23. Single or multiple copies of this article are
available for a fee from The Haworth Document Delivery Service [1-800-HAWORTH, 9:00 a.m. - 5:00 p.m.
(EST). E-mail address: docdelivery@haworthpress.com].

A SOCIO-HISTORICAL CONTEXT

Colonial Family Ethic

American women's transition from governmental assistance to work is rooted in the English Elizabethan Poor Laws of colonial times, when poor men and women were required to work in workhouses. This was called "indoor relief working to earn one's benefit" (Abramovitz, 1996; Gowdy & Pearlmutter, 1993; Rose, 1996). In colonial times, little sympathy was felt for the able-bodied poor, as settlers were bound by Calvinist ideology of hard work, which viewed idleness as synonymous with sin. Violating the colonial work ethic could result in being sent to a house of correction or the workhouse. Free white women were expected to marry, reproduce, manage the household, and be man's domestic subordinate.

In the Seventeenth Century, marriage was at the core of the family ethic. Colonial women were to acquire a husband and family and work in the home; these women who followed the family ethic were called "helpmeets" (Abramovitz, 1996). Motherhood was viewed as an essential task. The economy survived on subordinate labor, and female slaves were forced to work outside of their homes and outside of the family ethic. Race, class, marital status, and degree of servitude shaped women's experiences, given that colonial settlers brought women to the colonies as wives, servants, and slaves for their productive and reproductive labor. Poor women, by nature of their circumstances, confronted the family ethic and turned to the available forms of public relief. However, the powerful colonial laws regarding the poor looked to the rules and regulations of the family ethic to evaluate which women deserved relief. Because of their situation, they were not considered deserving of relief, yet, interestingly, white widows were considered deserving (Abramovitz, 1996; Rose, 1996).

Industrial Family Ethic

At the turn of the Eighteenth Century, great societal change occurred in response to the development of capitalist production. With the new economy, production became gender segregated. During the colonial period, women had carried out economically productive tasks in the home side-by-side with their male breadwinner. Now, however, the breadwinner was expected to work outside the home for wages, and the woman's place was in the home, caring for the children. The industrial family ethic clearly separated the roles of men and women, preventing women from paid labor outside the home (Abramovitz, 1996).

Women who were poor, of color, or who lacked a breadwinner had to work outside the home and were denied the opportunity to comply with the family ethic. Free black women, who had limited marriage possibilities due to a demographic shortage of black men and/or having the most menial jobs, headed their own families. As the century progressed poor women increased in numbers, and a new set of punitive ideas regarding the causes of poverty and the treatment of poor women emerged. Women who were out of role, poor and undeserving were punished with work in mental institutions, poor houses, and often separated from their children who were removed from their care because of poverty. Towards the turn of the nineteenth century, leaders of public aid and institutional care realized that it was best for children who had been removed from the homes of poor mothers to be placed instead back in their families or in a foster setting. At the beginning of the twentieth century, this problem was addressed by Mother Pensions, which provided the aid to keep a family together. However, the women who received this aid had to be considered deserving and fall within the broad domain of true womanhood bound by the family ethic (Abramovitz, 1996; Rose, 1996).

Progressive Period

Progressivism, the period between 1896 and World War I, was a cauldron of social shifts, with few experiencing great wealth but many more experiencing miserable poverty. It was a time of tremendous social reform to improve wages and working conditions, women's rights, health insurance, and pensions, and to end child labor. A kinder understanding of poverty emerged at this time: rather than attack the undeserving nature of the individual, poverty was blamed on the "social evils" beyond the control of the individual (Abramovitz, 1996).

To avoid poverty, women were moving into the workplace, but it was felt that a mother's employment negatively affected her children's development. Working mothers, both black and white, were blamed for juvenile delinquency and any other social or psychological childhood problem. Poor working mothers faced stringent barriers in trying to find childcare. Nurseries had strict eligibility requirements, and less than 40 nurseries in the country accepted black children. With the implementation of Mothers Pensions in the early twentieth century to care for children at home, the state began its role of overseer of family life and regulator of women's paid and unpaid labor (Abramovitz, 1996; Rose, 1995).

Modern Welfare State

Just prior to the Great Depression, public assistance was considered the responsibility of state and local governments and private organizations, but with the Great Depression came the need for many to be provided with subsistence as a substitute for the labor market that had fallen apart. Aid to Dependent Children (ADC, enacted in 1935 was an entitlement given to 88% of the families already receiving benefits because the father had died (Koon, 1997). By 1977, over 80% of the Aid to Families with Dependent Children (AFDC) consisted of divorced, separated, deserted or unmarried parents, with most of the remainder having incapacitated and unemployed fathers. With the lack of available jobs for male breadwinners, families faced desertion by the father and women struggled to find sex-segregated jobs; hunger and despair abounded. Black domestic workers who had lost their jobs set up a "slave market" on the streets, waiting for white women who needed their services for the day. Prostitution crossing all ethnic and racial lines became prominent (Jones, 1987; Rose, 1996). Although women's participation in the workforce increased during the Great Depression, public opinion voiced concern that women belonged at home, and corporations and government agencies began to terminate the employment of married women.

Post World War II

Government work programs after the World War II era were characteristically punitive and mandatory. Whenever their labor was needed, women on welfare were made available to work through "employable mother" policies. Aid to African-American women was denied at times of high seasonal demand for agricultural workers. Policies called "suitable home" and "substitute father" were designed to keep poor, mostly black women who had had children outside of marriage off the relief rolls. Poor women of color had only one recourse–to enter wage labor or marriage. By the 1960s, relief policies once again became more flexible for poor women (Rose, 1995).

Since the 1960s, women moved into the labor force in unprecedented numbers due to economic necessity. Some mothers chose welfare over work for a variety of reasons related to changes and trends in employment, family life, and adequacy of human capital (education and employable skills) (Abramovitz, 1996; Gerson, 1985; Koon, 1997). In 1962, Congress instituted social services to prepare welfare recipients to return to work and become self-sufficient. Federal welfare-to-work initiatives began with the Community Work and Training Program, which allowed states to require AFDC recipients to work off their benefit. In 1967, the Work Incentive Program (WIN) began with the goal of training all employable AFDC recipients for work, but in the early 1970s the focus shifted to job search and immediate employment (Koon, 1997). In the 1980s came the 1981 Budget Act, which restricted relief to the poor, followed by the Family Support Act of 1988, which focused on mandated work programs designed to make the poor earn their relief benefit while working in programs that were geared towards training and investing in human capital (Miller, 1990; Nathan, 1993; Rose, 1995).

All of these above-mentioned programs included the component of training to prepare for employment. However, training initiatives for TANF recipients is not included in the agenda of the 1996 Personal Responsibility and Work Reconciliation Act. Today, the TANF requirements regarding work and work related programs assert quick job preparation and placement strategy rather than a workforce investment strategy (Perlmutter, 1997).

Gueron and Pauley (1991) conducted extensive research evaluations on the effectiveness of training programs for welfare recipients in 13 states. While they found differences among the programs, their overall findings indicated that almost all the programs led to earnings gains. Earnings were sustained for at least three years after program enrollment, and public investments in a range of the programs were more than returned in increased taxes and reduced welfare payments. Interestingly, the most consistent and largest earning gains were made by the moderately disadvantaged. The researchers also found that mothers with young children had the most difficulty making the transition to work. These evaluation studies examined quantitative program outcomes and lacked qualitative data indicating the perspectives of welfare participants in the training programs. The effectiveness of mandated work programs to help poor mothers with young children needs further investigation to meet the needs of these families (Wittman, Staham, & Rhoades, 1997; Wittman, 1998).

Interaction Between Barriers to Work and Self-Sufficiency

Researchers and theorists have been interested in understanding how poor single mothers who are either welfare reliant or earning low wages survive when faced with barriers to employment (Berrick, 1995; Collins, 1994; Edin & Lein, 1997; Jones, 1987; Mink, 1998; Polokow, 1993; Rank, 1994; Schein, 1995; Sidel, 1996; Stack, 1974; Wittman, Staham, &

Rhoades, 1997). Ethnographic, oral history, and in-depth interview studies, combined with empirical data, have described the lives of poor women raising families, receiving welfare, and/or working in low-wage jobs (Berrick, 1995; Edin & Lein, 1997; Rank, 1994; Rhoades & Wittman, 1997; Schein, 1995; Stack, 1974). Such studies provide a foundation for research that underpins this dissertation.

Kinship Systems

In her seminal ethnographic study "All Our Kin," Carol Stacks (1974) investigated three central concerns of poor black families living in the Chicago Flats. She particularly examined the manner in which people are recruited into kin networks, the relationship between household composition and migration patterns, and the relationship between reciprocity and poverty. She began her research as an outsider–a white female–but she was able to enter the setting through a woman informant who was also a welfare recipient. This informant introduced her to two families with whom Stack eventually lived for three years and became accepted as a special insider, "White Caroline."

Findings showed that these poor black families survived poverty through a richly complex system of kinship: individuals who were related and individuals who were not formed intricate exchange networks that linked multiple domestic units and permitted elastic household boundaries with lifelong bonds with three generation households. Loyalties and a value system of internal sanctions maintained the bonds between members. Social controls within the kinship networks protected women from marriages because they could be destructive to the kin network. Any member of the kinship network that faced separation from the group through marriage or family also risked being marginalized from the generosity and exchange that helped maintain socioeconomic survival. This cultural system required sacrificing upward mobility and marriage, as well as moving away from kin, as a resilient structural adaptation for surviving poverty. Stacks' research provides a profound understanding of the coping strategies inherent in what she calls a "docile impoverished class" (p. 128) that is needed to maintain the present economic system with a low-wage labor pool.

Mental Health in Low Income Women

Another study conducted in the 1970s examined the relationship between stress and depression in low-income women and the effects on the parent-child relationship (Belle, 1994). The Stress and Family Project, spearheaded by Marcia Guttenberg, targeted interventions that would protect the mental health and function of mothers and their families. Belle (the project director) and her research team conducted a small-scale but intensive study of 43 women and their children. Over several months, participants were interviewed once or twice a week in their homes about various aspects of their life, including mental health issues. An observer also recorded six half-hour sessions of parent-child interaction, interviewed the children about the parent-child relationship, and then interviewed the mother about the relationship, parenting practices, and philosophy. The findings of the overall study suggest that the coping strategies for women varied dependent upon the circumstances surrounding their poverty. It was found that an individual who grows up in poverty is more at risk of being unable to leave poverty, whereas a middle-class individual who falls into poverty has a better chance of becoming self-sufficient because of better social resources.

As one of the researchers, Belle interviewed two women, one African American and one Caucasian. Belle found that the African-American mother had positive internal coping resources, such as a sense of humor and love for her children; however, she faced the personal barriers of alcoholism and the social barrier of having no kin with any resources that could benefit her. Although her kin and friends could provide emotional support and child-care, she was the one who provided material resources for her relatives.

Unlike Stacks' participants, this individual did not benefit from the kinship network system of reciprocity and material exchange that existed in the Flats. Similarly, in the Flats, kinship members stayed together in the community because moving away was viewed negatively. Thus, Belle had assumed that staying a long time in one's community was a positive strategy, but this African American participant who lived in a housing project in a crime-ridden neighborhood taught Belle that that was not a good thing. However, Belle's white participant, with whom she identified, had a different set of coping strategies that included a sense of entitlement and strong social resources. Thus, Belle found that to understand a woman's poverty circumstance, it is essential to assess race, ethnicity, class, gender issues, education, and discrimination experiences. Yet, establishing these categories beforehand may possibly prevent a participant from telling her story in her own words, as well as lead the participant to provide answers that please the interviewer rather than to follow a natural narrative course.

Getting Off the Edge

In 1980, Rank (1994) began to collect data for a broad quantitative/ qualitative study (*Living on the Edge*) that examined the experiences of individuals on welfare, starting with initiating the welfare process to getting off the rolls. The study sample represented the poor people of the United States rather than an underclass inner-city population, for it included female-headed families, couples, men, women, and the elderly. Rank (1994) interviewed 50 families on public assistance and also separately conducted fieldwork by visiting social service welfare agencies. The open-ended and semi-structured interviews lasted one-and-one-half to three hours and were conducted in the participant's home. Rank wrote field notes and took photographs after he received the participant's consent.

Data was collected at different times during a ten-year period. Changing socio-political forces and trends over that period may have affected individual circumstances and reasons for falling into poverty. However, Rank found that individuals on welfare are like all other individuals with similar American values regarding work and family. Faith, resilience and determination were the dominant coping strategies among the welfare recipients. Barriers to self-sufficiency were multi-layered, personal, social, and economic.

Rank found that welfare recipients faced severe economic hardship and psychological stigma. Relations within and outside the family were a constant source of pressure. Finding great diversity among different household types, Rank notes that welfare needs to be looked at in its broadest context. He views structural vulnerability as the primary challenge to poverty, that poverty is a problem of structural class differences rather than a work ethic or motivation problem. Individuals who face a crisis such as unemployment, illness, incapacitated young children, lack of personal resources and human capitol (education, marketable skills, training) or economic assets will have a more difficult time preventing a downhill slide into poverty. Rank questions why some people lack human capitol to begin with and relates this to the condition of social class reproducing itself.

Oral Histories of Poverty

In 1995, Berrick (1995) and Schien (1995) conducted qualitative studies to explore women's experience of welfare. In an earlier quantitative study, Berrick had found great diversity in child-care patterns and changes in family life of 400 poor women in the GAIN program in

California (Gilbert, Berrick, & Meyers, 1992). To obtain more detailed accounts of welfare-reliant women's experiences, she then conducted her 1995 qualitative study of five oral histories, *Faces of Poverty.* She conducted in-depth interviews in participants' homes (lasting up to six hours) and informal participant observation. Berrick reports that in some cases friendship occurred, but she does not explain how she dealt with her feelings, bias, or trustworthiness. Once again, Berrick found great diversity among welfare-reliant women. Barriers to self-sufficiency ranged from falling into poverty from unexpected circumstances, illness, and low-wage labor to drug histories, mental health issues, histories of sexual and physical abuse, and domestic and neighborhood violence.

Faces of Poverty stands out from other studies in its focus on the developmental transitions having an impact on the individual's psychological well being. In her analysis of the women's narratives, Berrick draws out themes of conflict in relationships with men and family, motivation, and psychopathology and sexual abuse that interfere with poor women achieving self-sufficiency. She concludes the diversity among these women demands that each woman's issue receive an individual response. Some women have job skills and do not need job training, others have major needs due to personal characteristics and environmental conditions, and still other women need individualized services as well as close case management to ensure the healthy development of their children.

Four Underlying Circumstances

Schien (1995), a board member of Survivors, Inc., and a member of the Job Training and Partnership Industry Council, became aware of the issues affecting low-wage workers receiving some public assistance. She decided to examine poor women's work issues within the context of their life histories and social circumstances. She interviewed 30 women receiving some form of public assistance and who had some work experience. The semi-structured, open-ended interviews ranged from 60 to 90 minutes. Schien's sequential interview protocol moved from demographics and work experience and then to past and present life experiences. She found four primary factors that underlie women's circumstances of poverty: absence of education and training necessary to qualify for a well paying job; betrayal by the mate (father of the children); negative childhood experiences; and non-supportive family influences. She also reports that each woman had a surprise circumstance that transformed her life, which may be linked to Denzin's (1997) notion of epiphany, also a transformative experience changing one's life. Schein's findings might have been more detailed had she conducted more than one interview per participant. More in-depth interviews might have led to linking barriers to self-sufficiency to the context of the surprise circumstances in the women's stories.

Stretching to Make Ends Meet

Edin and Leins' (1997) study of welfare-reliant women, *Making Ends Meet*, suggests that with the new time limits on welfare receipt, more single mothers will go to work. Although they will have more income than they had before, causing their poverty level to drop, they will have more expenses than they had on welfare, increasing material hardship. They found that, nationwide, mothers who are unskilled and semi-skilled face desperate economic and personal situations that they can seldom resolve satisfactorily. The researchers report that mothers relied on three basic strategies to bring income in line with expenses: work in the formal, informal, or underground economy; cash assistance from absent fathers, boyfriends, relatives, or friends; and cash assistance or help from agencies, community groups, or charities in paying overdue bills. Most mothers preferred to use networks rather than agencies, although networks were not always helpful in circumstances of friends having less resources or destructive relationships. These findings are concurrent with those of Stack (1974), Belle (1994), and Schein (1995). An additional finding of this study, however, is that mothers found the jobs they got did not make them any better off, and they felt that the transition from welfare to work would place them and their children at serious risk.

WELFARE REFORM IN THEIR OWN WORDS

In response to the PRA, the Women and Poverty Public Education Initiative conducted two survey studies in Wisconsin: In *Our Own Words: Mothers' Perspectives* on *Welfare Reform* (Wittman, Statham, & Rhoades, 1997); and In *Our Own Words. Mothers' Need for Successful Welfare Reform* (Wittman, 1998). The results of the examination of questionnaires completed by 740 welfare-reliant women suggest the emerging needs of family-supporting jobs, child-care, and education. Circumstances that led to poverty included single motherhood, inability to find a job, divorce or separation, job loss, and illness. Barriers to self-sufficiency were reported to be related to low wages, inadequate job skills, inadequate or affordable child care, no medical insurance, inadequate or no child support, ineligibility for social services, and abusive relationships. Although these findings provide general themes that validate previous studies, they do not add a greater dimension to these themes, except to point out the great need for childcare and higher wages.

INTERACTION BETWEEN WORK, FAMILY ROLE STRAIN, AND PSYCHOLOGICAL WELL-BEING: MOTHERWORK

Themes of survival, power, and identity are connected with mother work (reproductive labor) and psychological well-being in women of color (Collins, 1994). Mother work is characterized by survival, empowerment, and identity of both the individual and the community. Some women of color do this work only within the family, while others may work outside the home as well, and rely on "other mothers" (Collins, 1994, p. 216) or non-relation kin (Stack, 1974) to help care for families in order to strengthen the family and the community. Collins points out that for women of color, the work of motherhood is linked to the sociocultural concerns of their communities, while they independently search for autonomy. Conflict is perceived as outside the household, as women and their families engage in a collective effort to remain cohesive in a society that continually undermines family integrity.

COMPLYING WITH WORKFARE

Oliker (1995) explored how low-income single mothers on AFDC in Wisconsin became involved with paid work and how the structure of their personal lives shaped their personal actions. This study was conducted before time-limit sanctions for welfare assistance were implemented in the new welfare reform. The women interviewed in this study still had a choice between complying with Workfare programs or remaining at home to care for their children and work part-time off the books, as many did. Oliker found that when getting or keeping a job interferes with the psychological well-being of the children, mothers sometimes choose to lose wages and stay home. Low-income women are faced with low-wage jobs with high rates of turnover and unemployment, thus increasing the dependence on domestic networks for safety. Oliker points out that poor women are repeatedly faced with having to find work within a net of intricate family and community obligations in a society that cannot offer them sufficiently paid employment. The mothers interviewed by Oliker did not feel that Workfare policy always aimed to help them, nor did they think that working outside the home was always in the best interest of the family. Oliker notes that her findings cannot be generalized to all low-income women, particularly since the motivation for moral choice is not only economics.

Role Strain: Overload and Interference

Other studies explore how low-income women who have chosen to work face challenges managing the strain of work and family. In the 1980s, as the number of women in the labor force increased, work and family began to be viewed as interwoven spheres of life (Kelly & Voyandorf, 1985; Parasuramen & Greenhaus, 1997). Low-income women making the transition from welfare to work and attending mandated work programs face the potential strain of multiple roles (Rhoades, Statham & Wittman, 1997; Wittman, 1998). Kelly and Voyandorf (1985) state that working parents perform multiple roles, which requires time, energy, and commitment; hence, the cumulative demands of multiple roles can result in two types of role strain, overload and interference. Overload exists when the number of prescribed activities is greater than an individual can handle adequately or comfortably. Interference occurs when conflict between role expectations occurs and two different things have to be done at the same time. The level of role strain depends on the combined influence of the demands and resources associated with multiple roles. Role strain may be prevented or reduced when resources enabling individuals to cope with the demands associated with performing multiple roles are developed or provided. Available resources may include social, psychological, and human capital conditions. Sources of demands and coping resources associated with multiple roles can be categorized as individual, family-related, or work-related (Kelly & Voyandorf, 1985).

Poor single mothers participating in mandated work programs face all three of these categories of demand, while in many cases having inadequate coping resources, particularly in the area of human capital (Berrick, 1995; Rank, 1994; Schien, 1995; Wittman, 1998). Having a framework for work-family role strain provides an opportunity to identify stress that can lead to physical, emotional, and social problems for individuals and families (Kelly & Voyandorf, 1985; Pearlin, 1983; Warren & Johnson, 1995). Gerdes (1997) suggests a link between post-traumatic stress syndrome and long-term welfare-reliant individuals. She explains that a perceived punitive relationship between the welfare system, i.e., sanctions, repeated failure at sustained employment, lack of resources, may replicate prior dominant victimizing trauma-related relationships.

Another strain facing poor single mothers as they transition to work is the internalization of stigma related to welfare-reliance. Women who do not internalize stigma seem to have internal coping resources that enable them to take on an activist attitude and to work in collective protest regarding unacceptable conditions (Davis & Hagen, 1996).

Mythology of Model Families

The literature consistently describes single mothers with preschool-age children as having the most difficulty managing the multiple roles of work and family (Campbell & Moen, 1992). Single mothers who have been influenced by the family ethic may experience the pressure of meeting the expectations of the mythological two-parent family as interference impacting psychological well-being. Poor working mothers face challenges managing time, money, and energy shortages. There is the double-bind of experiencing feelings of failure of not living the normal two-parent family and meeting the demands of a single parent that requires a different set of behaviors (Quinn & Allen, 1989).

Stability of Situation

Goldberg, Greenberger, Hamill, and O'Neil (1992) found that the predictability of one's source of wages and how well wages meet one's needs are linked to the psychological well-being of women. They examined a range of factors associated with variations in a single mother's well-being, such as depression, role strain, and perceptions of her child's behavior. They found that an interface between work and family roles was important for a woman's well-being and perceptions of her children's behavior. Depression appeared to be more closely connected to the stability and resources in single mothers' lives. Role strain related to the time and energy demands of work and the level of support in the neighborhood. Single mothers' perceptions of their children were associated with the context of their lives, including divorce, newness to parenting, quality of work-life, and the points of intersection between work and family life.

Flexibility of Employment Hours

Warren and Johnson (1995) examined the relationship between work related coping resources and work-family role strain for a sample of 116 employed mothers with preschool age children in group day-care. The results of the study indicate that perceptions of the work environment, support, and supervisor flexibility, as well as the use of family-oriented benefits, are associated with lower levels of strain between paid work and family roles. While Workfare participants have no access to family benefits as a resource, the environment and supervisor flexibility can be enhanced to meet the needs of single mothers in mandated programs. The researchers outlined work-related demands that impact on the psychological well-being of single mothers: amount of work time, workweek scheduling, and long workweeks. In addition, psychological demands of the work-role with heavy workloads and pressure for output affect the lives of single mothers with young children.

Job-Family Role Strain

Examining job-family role strain in employed single mothers of preschoolers in Canada, Campbell and Moen (1992) found that strain was the most important predictor of emotional well-being. How mothers perceived maternal employment and the nature of the work experiences, as well as their personal meaning of work, were found to lead to different consequences for mothers in different circumstances.

Aguilar and Williams (1993) conducted an exploratory study examining the factors that minority women identify as contributing to their achievement and success. The study reported that ability and motivation are influenced by expectations, limitations and opportunities. Failure to achieve is associated with limited access to opportunities. The researchers interviewed 324 successful women who identified eight factors of success: achievement of goals, job satisfaction, self-esteem, education and skills and family support and stability, personal strength, ethnic-racial pride, and community and professional commitment. Culture, religious faith, and even racism and poverty were viewed as contributing to success. Although this study concurs with the previous literature, the voices of success and failure in the lives of low-income women still need to be heard.

Outcomes of TANF After 1996

Five years have passed since I interviewed the participants for this study. The reports discussed below have had a bearing on the impact on welfare reform since 1996 on the well-being of women in TANF and their children.

IMPACT ON CHILDREN

In its report *Children and Welfare Reform: Analysis and Recommendations* (2003), the Future of Children Organization notes that TANF families overall have done well since the inception of welfare reform. The organization found that poverty rates have declined and that, since 1996, many families have moved off welfare and into jobs. In August 1996, 4.4 million families had been receiving relief, whereas in September 2000, that number had declined by half–2.2 million. Many families leaving welfare and those who stayed on the rolls, according to the report, have faced serious barriers to employment.

The report also notes that welfare reform had positive impacts most often on school age children. Programs with the most positive impacts were those that increased family employment and income through earnings supplements without a mandatory work requirement. In addition, those programs also had small but significant impacts on the parenting practices of mothers who participated. It is important to note that the report states that programs resulting in families making no economic progress or experiencing a setback tended to negatively affect the children across all types of outcome measures. Since the attack on the World Trade Center on September 11, 2001, there has been a decline in economic resources among poor families. With over one million jobs disappearing since that date, especially in the low-wage areas of manufacturing, services, and transportation, poor families face even greater obstacles transitioning from welfare to employment.

Both Negative and Positive Effects

The study *Consequences of Welfare Reform: A Research Synthesis* (Grogger, Karoly, & Klerman, 2002), supported by the Rand Child Policy Project and conducted as part of Rand's Labor and Population Program, attempted to understand how welfare policies affect welfare-related outcomes. Synthesizing the current knowledge by examining numerous studies, Rand researchers found that welfare reform can have both negative and positive effects on children that may also vary with the child's age. The most favorable effects were associated with financial work incentives that result from a combination of welfare and work. Whereas work requirements were not indicated to have positive or negative impacts on children, they did have an unfavorable impact on adolescents. Blum and Francis discuss the need for research in several domains in their report *Welfare Research Perspectives: Past, Present and Future* (2002).

The authors found that more information is needed on the status of infants and toddlers and adolescents, particularly in light of the research that suggests some negative effects of welfare reform on youth. They note how several studies have shown that whereas most children have not been harmed by changes in welfare policy, children in households where income is supplemented when work is mandated have shown improved outcomes. When examining research on child outcomes, the authors suggest further study on the effects of work requirements for parents of adolescents and on the role of after-school programs on behavioral cognitive measures.

IMPACT ON HARD-TO-SERVE POPULATIONS

Blum and Francis (2002) also pay attention to other domains particularly pertinent to this study–the hard-to-serve populations that include disabled individuals and urban populations. The authors suggest that demonstrations to test models for serving those with multiple difficulties will help guide policymakers and practitioners toward creating productive programs. Studies of parents or children in families with a disabled individual reflected that parents or children may need assistance in coping. TANF families may be headed by parents who are mentally ill, developmentally disabled, physically disabled or physically ill.

Blum and Francis also looked at the research of TANF participants in urban areas and found that lack of affordable housing, greater cost of living, and higher crime rates, plus such barriers to employment as inability to access the job market and lack of education, may all contribute to slower TANF caseload declines in urban areas. Understanding the needs of low-income workers and responding to the barriers faced by more vulnerable individuals is a challenge (p. 13).

IMPACT ON ADOLESCENTS

An important study on the impact of welfare reform on adolescents was conducted by the Manpower Demonstration Research Corporation (Kaufman, Duncan, Gennetian, Knox, & Vargas, 2002) found that welfare policies have consistently unfavorable effects on adolescent school outcomes. Research synthesis of 8 studies of 16 programs reflects that school performance suffered and grade repetition increased among adolescents whose mothers were randomly assigned to the new work-promoting programs. The researchers declare that the impacts, although small on average, are statistically significant and merit the attention of federal and state policymakers who shape the course of welfare reform.

The Association of Maternal and Child Health Programs is concerned about the poor health of economically disadvantaged families. Their hope is that state welfare programs can take a vital role in mitigating hardships these families experience. Their document "Principles to protect the health interests of women, children, youth and their families" was created in response to the reauthorization of TANF in 2002 (Peterson, 2002). One of the ten principles, Principle 3, relates to the problems of adolescents examined in my study: "Promote the creation of positive youth development programs that reduce teen risk factors and give youth the foundation for a productive future." AMCHP had found that recent evaluations of welfare to work programs showed that adolescents were adversely affected the more parents worked. It was found that lack of supervision leads to adolescents being more likely to engage in risky behavior. They point out that, except for sexual behavior, teens are routinely ignored in public policy, a perspective that will be studied in the participants of my research.

doi:10.1300/J004v23n03_02

Chapter 3

Preparing for the Journey

SUMMARY. In this chapter, I first explain my research stance, which reflects how I became interested in this study, as well as the personal perspective and professional background that I bring to the study, which may clarify how I may hear and listen to the participants and face biases that emerge (Ely et al., 1997; Tedlock, 1995; Van Manen, 1990). Next, I describe the research setting, the participants, and the methods for recruiting the participants. Finally, I outline the research procedures, data collection, data management, analysis, methods to achieve trustworthiness, presentation of the findings, negative analysis, and preparatory study. doi:10.1300/J004v23n03_03 *[Article copies available for a fee from The Haworth Document Delivery Service: 1-800-HAWORTH. E-mail address: <docdelivery@ haworthpress.com> Website: <http://www.HaworthPress.com> © 2007 by The Haworth Press, Inc. All rights reserved.]*

KEYWORDS. Qualitative research, narrative, researcher's stance, interviews, data collection, data analysis

---

[Haworth co-indexing entry note]: "Preparing for the Journey." Greer, Ellen. Co-published simultaneously in *Occupational Therapy in Mental Health* (The Haworth Press, Inc.) Vol. 23, No. 3/4, 2007, pp. 25-39; and: *Women's Immersion in a Workfare Program: Emerging Challenges for Occupational Therapists* (Ellen Greer) The Haworth Press, 2007, pp. 25-39. Single or multiple copies of this article are available for a fee from The Haworth Document Delivery Service [1-800-HAWORTH. 9:00 a.m. - 5:00 p.m. (EST). E-mail address: docdelivery@haworthpress.com].

Available online at http://otmh.haworthpress.com
© 2007 by The Haworth Press, Inc. All rights reserved.
doi:10.1300/J004v23n03_03

OVERVIEW

This study was conducted using qualitative methods (Bogdan & Biklin, 1982; Ely, Vinz, Downing, & Anzul, 1997; Van Marten, 1990; Wolcott, 1994). Qualitative methods are suited to the inquiry of women's experiences to capture the bristling web of meaning in voice, emotion and action in daily life through narrative stories (Aptheker, 1989; Bruner, 1990; Cortazzi, 1993; Polkinghorne, 1988; Watson & Watson-Franke, 1985).

Women's transitional experiences in preparation to enter the workforce can begin to be understood from a perspective of their culture through a framework of narrative meaning, which views lived experience in its context of temporality, and personal actions (Cortazzi, 1993; Polkinghorne, 1988). I conducted in-depth interviews with six women who were participating in a mandated work program. Understanding their narratives by linking everyday actions and events into episodic units of experience can give form to understanding meaning in their lives. Storytelling can offer a framework for understanding past and present events. Upon reflection of these experiences, the opportunity arises for planning future actions (Polkinghorne, 1988).

As Bruner (1990) states, narrative is a mode of organizing experience, "composed of a unique sequence of events, mental states, and happenings involving human beings as characters or actors" (p. 43). Meaning is found in the overall sequence as a whole. It is the sequence of the telling of the story that is important, not whether it is real or imaginary. Stories explicate meaning by their deviation from the ordinary in a form that can be understood.

Cortazzi (1993) explains that narrative is viewed as a "speech event" and that "ways of narrating" involve variations according to components of the narrative situation. These variations include the participants, the setting, purposes of telling, communicative key, and cultural norms (p. 100). The telling of the narrative may depend on many factors, such as the relationship that has been developed, the setting of the interview, the mood of the narrator, and the reason for the narrative being told. Cortazzi suggests that the researcher pay attention to the "cultural ways of telling and the relationship between narrative styles and the contexts of narration" (p. 101). That is how I listened and heard the narratives of the women in my study–TANF recipients who were in the mandated workfare program, meeting the work-related activity requirement at an urban nursing home. I was guided by an ongoing reflection of my responses, thoughts, and feelings, with an ethical awareness of the complex relationship that existed between myself as researcher and the participants (Denzin, 1997; Ely et al., 1997; Naples, 1996; Patai, 1991).

Researcher's Stance: Human Research Instrument

My interest in women who have been forced to make the transition from welfare to workfare came as an outgrowth of a work readiness group I was conducting for mothers in an urban family school-based clinic in the first year of my doctoral studies. Going into the school, I had unrealistic expectations about how such a program develops. I began with several theoretical models in mind and planned exercises to facilitate group interaction, all without any real sense of the women with whom I would be working, their cultural legacies, or their needs. This experience brings into focus Denzin's (1997) comments on interpreting social life: Persons, for instance, mistake their own experiences for the experience of others. These interpretations are then formulated into social programs that are intended to alter and shape the lives of troubled people . . . . But often the understandings that these programs are based upon bear little relationship to the meanings, interpretations, and experience of the persons they are intended to serve. As a consequence, there is a gap or a failure in understanding (p. 11).

I thought I had the knowledge to begin such a program for several reasons. Personally, I shared similar gender roles with the mothers at the school. I, too, was a mother of children in school and had struggled over the conflicts of home versus work all my adult life. Although I had made the transition to work early on, it remained a source of constant tension, and I felt empathetic with women who were considering this path. Growing up in an extended family, where grandmother, mother, and aunt transitioned to work at significant moments in their lives, I saw how the family served as a container for all the feelings that emerged in life situations, and when there were disruptions in this unity, individual members suffered. I realized that I might still have had feelings of wanting to impose my values of family life onto both the TANF participants in the research partnership, as well as on my responses to workfare policy, and I planned that, should this occur, I would write reflective memos and talk in my support group about my emerging thoughts.

Professionally, I have had many years of training and practice as a therapist in occupational therapy and psychoanalysis, and I carry within me a chorus of ideas called theories. My initial experience with the work readiness group was humbling. Sitting with a group of low-income mothers of various ages, I gave up my plan and asked them what they wanted from the group. Over the next several months, women took turns as leaders to teach a specific skill. I became part of the group and facilitated the meetings with my co-leader, the school-based family clinician who knew the mothers and their children. The women became my teachers, and they allowed me to eventually learn about their lives, and they mine, as we worked together in a quiet constructive way, creating objects for the holidays. It was when we became a community of women sitting around the table, drinking coffee, eating the homemade cake, and sculpting a dream with moist clay that the women began to express their concerns about the safety of their children walking through intermittent gunfire in the projects and the letters that were coming from the welfare office telling them they had to work to earn their benefit or be sanctioned for non-compliance. What would happen to their children if unsupervised or who would be appropriate to babysit? Even if they did go to work, how much could they earn if they did not speak or read the language well? They did not have the choice any longer to stay home or be involved with motherwork through volunteering in their child's school, maintaining supervision and safety for all the children, not just their own.

Sensing Crises

I sensed that these women were undergoing a crisis of emotional, social, and political circumstance, and it awakened me to a new perspective. It seemed unfair and unjust that the mothers were being deprived of the right and the time needed to determine what they and their families needed. These women wanted to work; they came to the work-readiness workshop to sort out their priorities and to develop strategies over time. Their roles as mothers, guardians, and students were being altered without anyone hearing their voices or asking for their involvement.

The stakes had changed. Women were moving into workfare rapidly, and I was meeting them in my occupational therapy clinic to which they were assigned. Forced and rushed into a program, they were part of 200,000 women in New York City faced with a transitional crisis. I began to wonder how the women were experiencing this critical circumstance and how it was affecting their lives. Having administered a mandated program in the early 1980s (United Cerebral Palsy of New York State), moving large numbers of Willowbrook residents into the community, I was aware that my reaction to the mandated circumstance of TANF mothers was biased from the perspective of being a mother. In the face of workfare, I identified with the TANF mothers rather than tapping into my previous experience as an administrator, considering the goals and mission of the workfare program to assist people to become self-sufficient. It became clear to me that learning about workfare within a socio-historical context was required as a lens to understand the location of welfare-reliant women in this transition.

Awareness of Transition: Time Pressure

Knowing how program recipients think and feel in order to shape, improve, and or make necessary changes seems essential to helping people become successful. My thinking on this TANF workfare circumstance led me to readings in the feminist, work and family, and qualitative research literature. I began talking with female workfare participants and workfare program directors, and I came to believe that women's voices needed to be heard collectively through narrative. This became even more important because, since the PRA (1996), TANF recipients were now facing a five-year time limit to transition to employment. I strongly felt research was needed to understand how TANF recipients make and experience this transition, as they are facing a time limit that has not occurred before in their experience of workfare programs. Thus, I began to formulate my ideas for my study.

Awareness of Privilege

Being white, middle-class, married, and employed, as well as having strong support networks, placed me in a privileged zone in the eyes of the women who participated in the research, which caused me discomfort in respect to the differences in our lives and made me aware that my assumptions and biases can interfere with my seeing, inquiring, and hearing.

The first interfering assumption is that I tended to think of women living in poverty as sometimes despairing and unhappy, and yet, as I discovered in the work-readiness group and with the workfare participants in the clinic, the women often transcend their difficulties through creative action, humor, friendship, and spirituality.

My Multiple Lenses

I look through multiple lenses that are biased by my professional training and life experiences, which can exclude the seeing of other aspects of experience and can also promote the creation of silent theoretical categories that may be used to constrain what I am seeing or hearing. An important aspect of my professional background as a therapist is that I work to be open-minded and free of any agenda, always aware that someone else's theory is lurking in the background of my thoughts, trying to push in. I concentrate on listening with a "third ear" to pick up the subtle nuances and feelings that have not been put into words (Reik, 1949). This way of knowing that I brought to this study was consistently examined through logs, memos, and talking with my support group, committee, and other consultants, who brought to light any biases or interfering assumptions that were blocking what I saw, heard, or felt. In addition, I brought myself to the research as an instrument, who, because of practicing as a therapist, was aware of the temptation of wanting to intervene therapeutically in the life of a participant. I was careful to stay within my stance of researcher as instrument, to be sensitive to what was going on without making judgments or interfering with the process.

I was inspired by Christiansen (1997), who stresses that it is unethical to solely become enmeshed in uncomfortable feelings that are about difference. Instead, it is necessary to use privilege to help women whose lives are marginalized. I realized that conveying women's experience of the mandated workfare program through narratives may shed light on some understanding of their lives in transition from their point of view and provide information that will help other women in this situation and provide policy makers with ideas for direction.

Nursing Home Workfare Environment

This study took place at an urban nursing home that accepts workfare participants for the work-related activity assignment. The nursing home is a 150 bed facility that provides medical, nursing, and rehabilitation services to residents that have been admitted from the surrounding neighborhoods and community hospitals.

The environment of the nursing home is geared to meet the needs of the residents who are primarily Afro-American, Caribbean, and Hispanic. The majority of staff share similar cultural heritages with the residents and share holiday and religious celebrations as ongoing activities in the facility.

The residents who are admitted to the nursing home have been diagnosed with a range of medical and psychiatric conditions, such as stroke, Parkinson's disease, chronic schizophrenia, depression, Alzheimer's disease, and other organic syndromes. Workfare participants, who are called "volunteers" in the nursing home, may be assigned to different departments. They may either provide care-related activities for the residents or perform clerical tasks to support the administration of departments.

I had worked as an occupational therapist for 10 years in this nursing home, where I had been responsible for directing the occupational therapy program. I had already left the nursing home, but I returned as a researcher to conduct this study. The workfare participants interviewed for this study were working with the activities, nursing, housekeeping, or other departments. I was unfamiliar with the workings of those departments. Because I had been familiar with the occupational therapy program and to reduce bias, I did not include participants in the study who had been assigned to the occupational therapy program.

I was sensitive to questioning my assumptions and presuppositions about the familiar and learned to be open-minded to an expanded lens of hearing and listening to narratives about the unfamiliar within the familiar environment (Ely et al., 1991). In my role as a researcher, I worked on the experience of being an outsider. I wrote analytic memos about my experience of being an outsider in light of my recent insider role within this familiar setting.

Six Workfare Mothers

The participants in this study included five single mothers and one married mother. At the time of the study, the women were between the ages of 18 and 45 and were all TANF recipients. They were participants of either the WEP, BRIDGE, or BEGIN programs and were fulfilling the requirement to perform work-related activity in exchange for their benefit. The nursing home assigned workfare participants to the volunteer program, within the activities department; these workfare participants are referred to as "volunteers" throughout the facility.

The participants were at different stages of the program, although four out of six had been in the program for two years, and they had multi-cultural backgrounds. Five had been on welfare for over five years, and the other woman for less than three years. While four participants had not completed high school, two had obtained a GED in the program. In need of economic support, these women had turned to the welfare system for assistance as young mothers. They had been notified by the welfare office to report to workfare to earn their benefit with the implementation of welfare reform in an urban setting.

Approaching Nursing Home Management and Workfare Mothers

The recruitment process required the cooperation of both the director and assistant coordinator of the activities department, who were responsible for the work-activity assignments of the workfare participants. After the study was approved, I was invited to a weekly meeting that the activities coordinator led for the workfare participants. There, I was to introduce myself and say, I know you have experience that can shed light on how the mandated program is preparing women for employment. Since I am a doctoral student interested in learning more about this experience in order to help women in this situation, I will need your support. I am studying at New York University, and I previously worked in this nursing home as an occupational therapist when I had the opportunity to work with the volunteers.

I was to present my research interest to the participants, give a broad overviewof the research activities, and ask them to see me after the group if they would like to participate in the study. I would also give them my office telephone number if they wished to think about it and reach me at a later date. Interest of participants to take part in the study would not be communicated to the activities departments to avoid the participants experiencing any pressure at the worksite.

Recruitment became more complicated than expected. I planned to include up to eight participants and to have a reserve list of additional participants for availability should any participants drop out. If more than eight participants signed up for the study, I planned to interview everyone for about 10 minutes and then select participants based on their interest and willingness to be part of the study. If less than eight signed up, I planned to have another group meeting with new workfare participants and would continue this procedure until there were enough participants. However, only six women ended up participating in this study. (See Chapter 4, which is devoted to entry to the field.)

When I met with the six workfare participants who had volunteered to be interviewed after three recruitment meetings, I went over in detail my research methodology and asked the participants where they would like to meet and if they had any questions about the research. I explained the audio taped interview and participant checking process and made it clear that the tapes would always be available for them to listen to, and that at the end of the study the tapes would be destroyed. Over the course of the study, the six participants never requested any portions of the audio-taped interview be deleted. Participants also decided the location of the interviews. All six were held in various locations within the nursing home, each where the individual participant felt comfortable.

After participants volunteered to take part in the study, I explained the interview process and the purpose of the consent form. (See Appendix A.) It was clear to the potential participants that they did not have to be part of the study, nor would there be any repercussions at the work related site or with TANF if they decided to withdraw. Furthermore, as participants in the study, they were assured that their names, workplaces, or any other identifying information would not be mentioned in the study or any subsequent publications. Small details, such as location, ages of children and gender, have been changed to protect the anonymity of the research participants. In addition, they were given a letter informing them of a doctoral advisement committee member to contact if they had any questions or concerns about the project. (See Appendix B.)

Conducting Interviews

This qualitative study involved audio taping and close observation during the interviews of TANF workfare participants who were assigned to work-related activities at an urban nursing home. I began the interview process after the New York University Human Subjects Committee approved my study and after the workfare participants gave me informed consent.

When I initiated the interview process with the participants, I discussed possible times and locations for the interview at the nursing home. Because the participants were initially guarded and did not want me to contact them at home about setting up a time for the interview, I made contact in person at the nursing home. During each interview, I let the participant know when I turned on the tape recorder. The tape recorder was acceptable at all the interviews by each participant and no one ever asked me to turn it off. I took no notes during the interviews.

I conducted interviews with one participant at a time. At the beginning of the first interview, I explained to the participant that I viewed her as my teacher and was interested in her experiences. Follow-up interviews, also conducted one at a time, occurred over the course of two to nine months to meet the convenience of the participants. This expanded time period also allowed me to follow the participant's progression of experiences and also gave me ample time to transcribe the interview. After each interview, I transcribed it into a text that became the data that I analyzed to understand the participant's perspective. Prior to beginning the follow-up interviews, I analyzed the transcriptions for new questions and understandings for the next interview. I studied pertinent parts of the transcription with the participant prior to the follow-up interview to obtain her view on what was said and whether any part needed clarification or expansion. After this had been checked, I proceeded with the follow-up interview. Each participant had at least two interviews; more were conducted when additional information or clarification was needed. At the second interview, I asked the participants if there was anything they wanted to learn from this experience. This study was expected to take between three to six months to complete. It took one year. This more realistic time frame allowed me to conduct as many follow-up interviews as I needed.

Field Logs and Analytic Memos

In addition to the interview transcripts, my working materials throughout the study were my field logs and analytic memos. Samples of each can be found in Appendix C. Field notes were kept on my observations of the setting and the interactions during the interviews. I kept a pad and pen with me at all times. When I was in the setting, I sometimes found a moment to leave and go to a private space and jot down some observations, or on my travels on the train, I wrote about my observations, as well as when I arrived home later in the day. However, I did not write in the presence of the participants.

Analytic memos were written at home or in my office on a laptop computer. The notes that I kept from my observations were incorporated into the memos and linked to the connections I made from the transcription data. The analytic memos reflected my ideas and feelings that emerged from the data and literature pertinent to the study as it progressed. The memos served as a continuous reflection in considering the initial research questions and also functioned as the "audit trail" of the research process.

I transcribed all the interviews and I reviewed each transcript against the tape for accuracy, as well as reviewed portions of the interview with each participant. After this, I began to incorporate the field note observations and then started coding and comparing the data with previous interviews and analytic memos.

Data Collection Interviews

Qualitative in-depth interviewing is a way to discover what others think and feel about their world (Denzin, 1997; Ely et al., 1991; Rubin & Rubin, 1995). The interview is a strategy to "gather descriptive data" in the words of the participants in order for the researcher to gain insight by hearing in the participants' own words their interpretations of "some piece of the world" (Bogdan & Biklin, 1982, p. 135).

Rubin and Rubin (1995) define three characteristic elements of qualitative interviewing that they view as a philosophical approach to learning. The first element encourages individuals to describe the world in their own terms. The second illuminates the research-participant relationship and the obligations on both sides. The third "helps define what is interesting . . . . what is ethical and helps provide standards to judge the quality of the research, the humanity of the interviewing relationship, and the completeness and accuracy of the write-up" (p. 2). Through the lens of this philosophical approach to learning, qualitative interviewing is a multi-layered transaction creating knowledge, mutual responsibility, and trustworthy scholarship. The process of the interview that generates knowledge is well described by Ely (1991) as "interwoven dances of questions and answers in which the researcher follows as well as leads" (p. 59). Van Manen (1990) views the interview as a means for "exploring and gathering experientially narratives that may serve as a resource for developing a richer and deeper understanding of human phenomenon" and that this comes about as a "conversational relation" develops between the research partners, enhancing the unfolding of meaning of an experience (p. 66).

I was aware that my role as research instrument in the interview process was to hear the participant's stories, to stay close to the participant's experience, and to ask questions to bring out the fullness of the experience. At the same time, I was aware of the purpose of the research questions and led with open-ended questions that maintained a sense of disciplined flexibility.

As described earlier, participant checking was an important aspect of the interview process, in refining and elucidating the participant's narrative, as well as refocusing on the research questions and making any needed changes as I gained more understanding of the participant's perspective.

Close Observation During Interviews

Close observation is a method of obtaining experiential material (Van Manen, 1990). I closely observed the interaction between myself and the participants during interviews, in the setting, and during any other phenomena that occurred. In addition, I closely observed when a participant invited me to participate in any aspect of her life experience. I was open to opportunities where I could observe the participant with her consent. I adjusted to whatever experiences the research required in participating and observing, while keeping the research goals in mind at all times. While I maintained a position of being as close to the experience as possible and as close as possible to my own reactions, I was aware of myself as a research instrument, moving back and forth to reflect on what I was seeing and hearing and feeling. Experiences that I observed were recorded in field notes at the end of the day at home or in my office. The field logs containing my transcripts, observations, and comments served as data for analysis.

Data Management of Logs and Notes

I used the field log to organize what I heard, saw, experienced, and thought during the course of the data collection (Bogdan & Biklin, 1982). I recorded my ideas, reflections, hunches, and any patterns I saw emerge in analytic memos. Field notes of my observations, analytic memos, and interviews served as my process to reflect on the research journey from the inception when I gained access to interviewing the participants. The written material assisted me in comparing and contrasting conceptual information, informing me of gaps and/or connections to be explored. The log challenged me through reflection to consider the ethical nature of the research partnership and how it was evolving and any changes that needed to be made in the methodology (Strauss, 1987).

My field logs were typed into a computer on Word Perfect 6. The design of the log provided large margins on both sides so that I could write comments on the sides. Each page was paginated and each line was numbered, which helped me to identify data in the analysis process. As I developed categories, subcategories and thematic statements, I created files on the computer and a cut-and-paste method in coded envelopes. The envelopes were considered my files.

Data Analysis of Categories and Themes

Data analysis is a way to "tease out what we consider to be essential meaning in the raw data" (Ely et al., 1991, p. 140). The recursive process of analysis guided me to focus and refocus the lenses through which I examined the data. In addition the recursive process of analysis helped me think about refining the research question if pertinent when I checked out emergent hunches with questions, insights, and ideas in conjunction with reading as I went along (Ely et al., 1991; Van Manen, 1990).

Polkinghorne (1988) notes that a goal for research into the production of meaning within narrative is to "produce clear and accurate descriptions of the structures and forms of the various meaning systems" (p. 161). To lift and distill the embedded meanings of experience in narrative, analytic procedures of coding, categorizing, comparing and contrasting categories, and identifying emerging patterns and themes are required (Ely et al., 1991, 1997; Strauss, 1987; Van Manen, 1990). To further open up the analysis to obtain the essence of meaning, various analytic techniques, such as metaphor analysis, layered stories, poetry, playlets and pastiche, can be created with the data (Ely et al., 1997).

Coding: Conceptualizing Categories and Their Relationship

Coding is a general term for conceptualizing data into categories and defining the relationship between categories (Strauss, 1987). I began line-by-line coding during the data collection phase by choosing portions of interview transcript text, field notes, and analytic memos to read over several times to obtain its essence of meaning. Then I wrote notes in the margins that consisted of my ideas, insights, and questions that related to the data I had just read. Next, I became aware of any changes or progressions in the meaning and made notations that divided the narrative "portioning meaning units" (Ely et al., 1991, p. 88; 1997, p. 88). The meaning unit may be found in a few words, a sentence, several sentences or paragraph. In the margins of the line of the meaning unit, I labeled what the meaning unit was about using only a few words.

Category Labels: Analytic Memos Reveal Linkages, Comparisons and Contrasts

After reviewing several portions of text and logs, I made a list of labels, grouped the ones that fit together, and found a label to head this group. Wolcott (1994) calls this labeling *binning*. Those labels that did not fit together were grouped independently. I looked for linkages, comparisons, and contrasts between labels. It is important that the label describes the meaning unit, even if it only occurs once. With the group of labels, I recursively repeated the process of reading text, notes, and memos. When I discovered new meaning units, I applied the defined labels. If the labels did not fit, I created new ones until I developed a "sensible organizing scheme" (Ely et al., 1991, p. 88). Labels that served as the coding process could be considered as categories when the labels fit the meaning units. As I moved through this procedure, I wrote analytic memos about the relationship between identified categories, which led to lifting categories to higher levels of abstraction (Ely et al., 1997; Strauss, 1987). In the writing of analytic memos, I found other connections that helped to distinguish emerging themes within and throughout the categories (Ely et al., 1997; Strauss, 1987; Van Manen, 1990).

Common Patterns/Themes Emerge as Stories, Playlets or Poems

Themes are statements that describe the essence of meaning in the data as I understand it and that make clear relationships between the categories. Thematic statements may express a central issue or concern about the participant's experience or may address key issues that may be common among several participants' experiences.

As I worked on coding and categorizing, I began to see patterns and themes emerge. To bring out the patterns and themes, I used various methods to discover what was going on. I considered writing a layered story to examine the multi layers of a participant's anecdote, developing a playlet to show the facets of experience, or writing a poem using the participant's words. Using these methods is a way of digging deep to bring forth the treasure of meaning and perspective (Ely et al., 1997).

Tables and Graphic Displays

Tables and graphic displays can be used to represent demographic information related to the participants. In this study, information was gathered about suggestions to improve workfare and barriers to employment. This information is represented in Table 1 (Chapter 7) and 2 (Chapter 11), respectively.

Trustworthiness and Credibility of Interviews and Narratives

I used several methods to work towards trustworthiness and credibility of the study. It is essential that the researcher aim to present the findings of the study that reflect the participants' experiences. To start with, I examined my own responses, thoughts, and feelings in several ways. Reflection was an ongoing process through writing analytic memos. I presented my reactions, as well as written analytic memos and data analysis, to a support group for their ongoing feedback. The support group was made up of members who were doctoral students in the fields of international education, recreation, and special education and who were going through the dissertation process. My committee also provided me the opportunity to raise difficult issues related to the trustworthiness and credibility of the study.

Participant Checking of Themes: Responses and Viewpoints

At the end of the study, when I was writing up the findings, I met again with five of the participants who could be reached to review some of the themes or other creations I had developed to see how they resonated with them. One of the participants who left the program several months before the end of the study could not be reached.

I was interested in each participant's response and point of view. If there was incongruence between the findings and the participant's reaction, I was prepared to consider how I had interpreted the data. Three participant checks were conducted at the nursing home and two took place at the homes of the participants during the summer. For the participants who had trouble reading, I read portions of a story or a poem. They were in agreement with my presentation. The participants' literacy levels varied. Those who could read were given excerpts to read. One participant said I had described her life, and another appreciated the way I described her home and life.

Negative Case Analysis

As I analyzed the data and developed themes, I looked for incidents or cases that challenged those themes. Alternative points of view were analyzed for context and explored in more detail by re-reading and re-analyzing and often retitling categories and bins (Ely et al., 1997). The relevance of this technique is in helping the researcher critically examine the findings and reanalyze them in light of negative cases that occur. This critical technique ensures that the final themes are as true to the data collected as possible. For example, negative case analysis emerged when analyzing how the participants fit the mandated program into their daily lives. For two of the participants, leaving the program was necessary for their perceived well-being. As another example of a negative case, five participants felt prepared for employment, but one did not.

Presentation of Findings:
Multiple Perspectives of Central Themes

In the presentation of the findings, I attempt to describe, analyze, and interpret the essence of meaning I found in the narratives of the participants' experiences. I attempt to show the multiple perspectives of the participants' experiences through my presentation of central themes that I uncovered. I compare and contrast different perspectives so that the reader can make connections to how those perspectives influence the participants' lives.

I create a conversation with the related literature. I discuss where my data are in agreement with the literature and where there is disagreement with other scholars and researchers. I explore the questions my data may raise about the experiences of women participating in the mandated work program.

doi:10.1300/J004v23n03_03

Chapter 4

Entry into the Field:
Can You Help Us Get a Job?

SUMMARY. In this chapter, I describe the nursing home setting of this study and my experience in recruiting the study volunteers, including the problems and resistance I had to overcome in gaining their permission to be interviewed. It should be noted that when describing the meetings, I refer to the volunteers generally as "Ms." or "Woman," as I had not yet gained their consent. When I refer to the volunteers as "the girls," it is in a specific context in relation to how their supervisors referred to them or how they were referring to each other. In subsequent chapters, I use pseudonyms for the volunteers. doi:10.1300/J004v23n03_04 *[Article copies available for a fee from The Haworth Document Delivery Service: 1-800-HAWORTH. E-mail address: <docdelivery@haworthpress.com> Website: <http://www. HaworthPress.com>* © *2007 by The Haworth Press, Inc. All rights reserved.]*

KEYWORDS. Recruitment, observation, gatekeepers, consent, welfare mothers

---

[Haworth co-indexing entry note]: "Entry into the Field: Can You Help Us Get a Job?" Greer, Ellen. Co-published simultaneously in *Occupational Therapy in Mental Health* (The Haworth Press, Inc.) Vol. 23, No. 3/4, 2007, pp. 41-56; and: *Women's Immersion in a Workfare Program: Emerging Challenges for Occupational Therapists* (Ellen Greer) The Haworth Press, 2007, pp. 41-56. Single or multiple copies of this article are available for a fee from The Haworth Document Delivery Service [1-800-HAWORTH, 9:00 a.m. - 5:00 p.m. (EST). E-mail address: docdelivery@haworthpress.com].

NEW ROLE: CROSSING A BORDER

Entering the nursing home as a researcher in July, 1998, I was filled with the anticipation of a novice who has no idea that all one's plans can go away. Perhaps it is best that I began this study with such naiveté, for had I known what was to come, I might have given up before I started. Returning to the nursing home in a new role with the purpose of learning about the volunteers' experience required a letting go of old expectations and satisfying roles, assumptions, habits, and relationships so that I could be open to whatever lay before me.

Given this reality of crossing a border, feeling completely other and strange in an environment that was once but no longer familiar, I was faced with surviving in a culture that demanded I relate to others in ways yet unknown to me. Over time, it is this painful experience of being an outsider and feeling like an intruder that brings me to understand and connect with the volunteers.

When I began the study, I was just becoming familiar with workfare philosophies, policies, and program models. I assumed that welfare reform was about moving people from welfare to work. Perhaps that is why I assumed that the mandated program was going to help the participants move into the workforce, and that is why the participants expected that they would be given jobs. Peck (2000) states that workfare tends to keep the participant in a state of job-readiness–close to a job, but not quite there.

There are four models of workfare: market, local-state, community sector, and human capitol (Peck, 2000). The market model is known to move people quickly into the work force. The community sector model is designed to offer full-time training in a particular skill to benefit a community program. The human capitol model provides full-time education and training. The group of women I interviewed at the nursing home were participating in the local-state model, designed to provide work activities in exchange for the recipient's welfare check. This model incorporated two days of school per week for individuals without a GED.

The nursing home had no formal training or goal-setting program for the workfare participants. Once accepted by interview into the nursing home's volunteer program, the workfare participants were given the organizational title of "volunteer" and a general orientation of "do's and don'ts." The paradox here is that although they were labeled *volunteers*, the participants were in a coercive situation. As one study participant said, *"If you call me volunteer, I won't answer won't answer. Call me 'intern' and treat me like a professional."* Informally, the participants were known as "the girls" within the organization, and they often referred to each other that way, as well. The formal and informal titles placed the participants on the lowest level of the organizational hierarchy, that is, "unpaid worker." In any event, most nursing home staff, as well as the alert residents and their visitors, recognized the volunteers' status as welfare recipients by their badges that identified them, pinned on their clothing.

Low-skilled nursing home employees were threatened by the presence of the volunteers (Ensetlem, 1997), fearing that their employer might replace them with this free workforce. Resentment toward the volunteers was communicated through demeaning remarks and social exclusion by various levels of staff. A counterbalance to this negative behavior was the mentoring provided by the nurses and supervisors, who took an interest in the volunteers' capabilities.

THE NEIGHBORHOOD:
COMMUNITY AND NURSING HOME IN THE "HOOD"
OBSERVATION ON A FRIDAY MORNING:
PAINTING A PICTURE

It was summer, hot and sticky. A month had already passed since I had begun my research visits. Getting off the bus on a Friday morning a block away from the nursing home, I wondered how the surrounding neighborhood influenced the meaning of the nursing home for the volunteers. Ann Lamott (1995) became my guide. In *Bird by Bird*, she writes how important it is to observe for a long time so as to get past the initial stimulation and distractions–to find out what is underneath.

On the bus stop corner is a Jamaican restaurant. On the other side of the street (a major thoroughfare) and directly opposite, nestled between tenements, is Kingston Chicken, another frequently visited restaurant. The subway entrance next door to Kingston Chicken makes for a busy corner.

As I crossed the side street, a white van advertising ASPCA Animal Protection in bright red letters pulled up to the corner. On this day, it appeared as if all the neighborhood stray dogs had vanished. Usually, several weathered dogs roamed the avenue, finding nourishment outside of the many restaurant kitchens along the blocks that I walked. Often they stayed near the back of the nursing home, resting or restless until they find something to eat.

On this day, as I walked down the block, I spotted a small lot behind a tall twisted metal fence. Standing in the middle of the lot was a gutted-out yellow school bus. Above an opening in the rear of the bus was a sign that read, "gifts here." A man and woman stood alongside the bus, holding and possibly exchanging foodstuffs; the friendly vibe-intonation in their voices suggested an amiable conversation. Walking by, I noticed a medical clinic for welfare recipients across the street. Down the next block was a new modern HMO for individuals in the neighborhood who had private insurance.

At the end of the street was a newly refurbished restaurant. I remembered when it had been a Chinese take-out only a few months before. An armed robbery had left its glass windows smashed, riddled with bullets, but the building had soon been restored with a new bulletproof take-out window to protect employees. It is possible that a feeling of safety had never been rekindled, for the restaurant had remained empty and eventually was replaced by the new family style eatery with curtained windows and a colorful entrance.

I could see the nursing home across the street, a modern brick and glass building. Nobly situated on the corner, it is the home for the community's vulnerable ill elderly. Here, staff members' informal rules state that no form of violence is tolerated. Any petty crime requires a serious investigation, and insulting someone's cultural legacy leads to the person's being cast out on his or her heels. My past experience working in this environment, coupled with my present observation of the volunteers hanging out together in front of the building protected by a tall iron fence, made me aware that individuals thrive from feeling safe in this space. They smoke, joke around, and complain to one another with ease.

In the open playground across the street, beyond the protective fence, bullets fly from time to time. Betty and Esther, volunteers who were to become study participants, later explained that death by gunshot in the neighborhood is part of their everyday experience. "It's no big *deal,*" they responded in unison. I was surprised to discover that violence in the volunteers' lives was usually reported without any feeling. In the safety of the nursing home, the volunteers were free to develop relationships, consider their situation in workfare, and commiserate about their lives. In time, I would learn more about their feelings and attitudes in the face of fear and uncertainty.

GATEKEEPERS: TOO BUSY TO BE AT THE GATE

Camilla Hernandez was the Director of Volunteer Activities at the nursing home, and her staff consisted of one full-time employee, Dorothea Smith, who had worked her way up the ranks from workfare and served as her assistant. Camilla's secretary, Susan, and a number of volunteers were from the mandated workfare program. Camilla was responsible for administering the volunteer program, and Dorothea assisted her in monitoring the paper work and providing on-site supervision.

Both Camilla and Dorothea were familiar with my study from when I had worked at the facility, and they offered their support, including helping me recruit volunteers for the interviews. Having had a collegial relationship with them from our many years of working together led me to assume that I would have a smooth transition in my new role as a researcher. However, even with their support, the transition was difficult. I had believed Dorothea would be at the recruitment meetings to introduce me, but given the demands of her job, her absences from the three meetings I conducted left me in the raw position of the volunteers wondering, "Who is this person?"

Group Meetings of Potential Interview Participants

The meetings began in August. I was eager to get started. It took several months of disappointment and uncertainty before I obtained any consents to begin the interviews. However, with each meeting, I began to learn more about my question of "what was underneath." I also learned not to give up on the volunteers or myself. We were striving to find an acceptable balance where we could enter into a safe relationship, and that took time. The following excerpts from my field logs illustrate the recruitment process.

FIRST MEETING WITH AN APPREHENSIVE GROUP OF "THE GIRLS"

I was sitting in the recreation office waiting for Dorothea to come downstairs so that we can go to the meeting together. Susan, the secretary, was sitting at the desk, monitoring questions of residents and volunteers as they come in and out of the office. William, a resident, munching on candy, wheeled into the office and began to interview me about my latest plans. He knew me as his previous therapist.

The phone rang. Susan picked it up.

Susan: *That was Dorothea. She said you should go upstairs to the dayroom. "The girls" will come down for a meeting.*

Camilla explained that the volunteers are called "girls" as a way to distinguish them from the staff. Yet she sees it as friendly.

I went up to the second-floor small dayroom, across the floor from the large dayroom. Walking into the sunny space with glass windows facing the courtyard garden, I noticed the layered leaves of the magnolia tree reaching towards the sky. Refocusing, I became aware of several residents sitting in the surround. Against the far left wall, Molly, squinched face, sat rigidly in her Geri chair, softened by the fluffy quilt that served as lateral supports and a comfortable landing for her arthritic arms and hands. Patti and Ina, the highest functioning ambulatory residents on the floor, sat opposite each other at the dining table in the center of the room. I joined them for several minutes to discuss the latest news of the 2nd floor.
A woman walked in.

Ellen: *Are you here for a meeting?*
Woman 1: *I'm here to clear the place for the meeting and get it ready.*

She wheeled Molly out of the room. I thought she looked like one of the volunteers. How did I make that assumption? She was wearing a nametag; she wore regular clothes rather than a uniform and had a noticeable look of disconnection. This particular look I learned later was specific to Agnes. After some time passed, two women came into the room. Together, we sat at the table in the far left corner, some distance from Patti and Ina. I thanked the women for coming.

Woman 1: *Others are going to come.*
Woman 2: *Yeah, but we don't know when.*

I told the women about the research. Woman 1 made no eye contact. She seemed removed and stayed silent. Woman 2 introduced herself as a mother of three children.

Woman 2: *I want to be paid for this work I want a good job. You don't know what this program does to a family I have three children. How can I get a good job? I want to be paid for this. I'm working for nothing.*
Woman 1: *(Silent while the other speaks. I sense her guardedness.)*

Shortly two more women entered the room and joined us at the table. As we talked and repeated the purpose of the research, another women in whites walked in. Her uniform suggested she was a nurse's aide. I learned that volunteers who worked for nursing had to wear a white uniform.

Woman 5.   *I am Ms. Dee. Dorothea asked me to come to this meeting*
              to see what is going on. (She stands up alongside the table
              with a vigilant presence that arouses a wave of anxiety)
Woman 3:   *What will I get out of this? I want to get something out of*
              this! I want something to happen. We keep going around
              in a circle.
All Women: *We're going around in a circle.*
Woman 4:   *Some things won't change.*
Ellen: *What would you like to get out of this?*
Woman 3:   *Jobs! We need jobs. Can you get us a job?*
Woman 4:   *Something has to happen. We keep coming back here,*
              and no-one gives us a job.

I explain the purpose of the research in relation to their concerns; however, I make it clear that I cannot find them jobs. This is disappointing to the women. We talked about the consent forms. The group becomes quiet. There are no questions. Then,

Woman 1:   *Could the consent form be signed with a different name?*
Woman 2:   *Maybe I would sign but I have to think about this.*
Ms. Dee: *O yes! This is something you have to think about.*

After discussing the details of where to bring the consent forms, I thanked everyone for coming, and all at once they got up to leave. I sensed that they were scared. Ms. Dee, who was sent to observe and determine the safety of the project for the volunteers, made her impression so strong that I did not hear from any of the volunteers. One of the volunteers left an empty envelope for me at the agreed upon spot the following week, making her refusal clear. I wondered if things would have been different if Dorothea were there.

SECOND MEETING WITH "THE GIRLS" AND A CONCERNED GATEKEEPER BEFORE THE MEETING

The next week I met with Camilla to go over my plans for a group meeting and to discuss my concerns about scaring the volunteers with signing consent forms. Camilla told me to leave that part up to Dorothea. It shocked me when she expressed her own suspicions that signing the consent form could lead to trouble:

Just leave that part to Dorothea. The women don't understand. They are used to getting so many forms from welfare and signing. (sigh) I hope this won't come back to haunt them.

I explained how the consent form protects the rights of participants. Camilla seemed more comfortable and talked to me about the volunteers:

A lot of "the girls" have husbands or boyfriends who are in jail, and they support them with the welfare check. They send them up $20 here and there to buy things, with the hope that when they come out they are going to support them again. These girls had everything. The man was a drug dealer on the streets and they had lots of money–houses, clothes, all the comforts, and the men are now in jail, and they hope when they get out they'll be taken care of again. "The girls" have no goals for themselves, nothing; they just wait for the day for the man to return. Then they'll have comforts. They can't put the money in the bank because they're on welfare, so they put it on their bodies, buy houses, all material things. They were rolling in money and had a good life.

Contradictions were taking shape. Camilla was saying that while the volunteers were on welfare, they were living very well on the economics of drug dealing. Now that their partners were incarcerated, the major source of income disappeared, leaving some of the volunteers meeting the requirements for welfare benefits.

Underneath Camilla's commentary was the message that the volunteers used the system when they did not need it. Her perception that the volunteers were without goals and aspirations did not match the perspectives I heard from the volunteers. Was this clash a symptom of some deeper misunderstanding between Camilla and the volunteers?

The phone rang. Camilla picked it up and then said:

Dorothea has the girls together. They're waiting for you in the second floor dayroom.

I got up to leave when Dorothea walked into the office. She was eating a pear, said a few words to Camilla and left to continue organizing the meeting. I had the hopeful impression that she was going to be there.

In the Dayroom: Collision of Voices

I walked into the dayroom. Six women were sitting around the room in a semi-circle. I recognized Woman 1 from the first group, who gave me no eye contact but asked if she could sign the consent form in a different name. My eyes went to the woman with a sleeping child on her lap. All the volunteers were focused on this pair, as well. While I slid into a seat, the conversation around me was a debate and exploration about whether or not it is all right to bring your child to work. *What are you going to do if there is no child-care? You gotta bring your kid!*

The conversation relaxed, so I asked if Dorothea were coming. Everyone said yes, so I sat quietly waiting. Time passed.

Why Are We Here?

The volunteers seemed to be getting uncomfortable. I told them it was because of me, and it looked like Dorothea wasn't coming. After explaining who I was and the purpose of the research, I stated that I wondered whether the work experience was preparing them for employment. Before my words ended, an outpouring reaction like a major chord occurred all at once. It was hard for everyone to separate out their own stories and wait a turn to speak. Collision of voices:

There are no jobs
This is a circle you go around over and over.
This is my third year here.
I go to job club twice a week. You read the newspaper.
Monday,Tuesday, and they say,
THE JOB IS TAKEN
I went to all the nursing homes in Farming Hill.
There are a lot of them run by the Jewish people.
And there are no jobs.
THERE ARE NO POSITIONS HERE.
They say you can't get into this place unless you have a family working here.

When everyone settled down, the room became quiet for a moment. One by one the volunteers said something about their individual concerns with workfare.

Ms. Adams: *This is the second time I am at this nursing home. My area is clerical. I have had years of office experience. When I lost my job, I had to go on welfare. Whenever I am given an assignment, I do a professional job. If there is an opening, I fill out the application. I never get hired. I am angry and wonder if a grievance can be filed and brought before the mayor.*

Ms. Barkley: *I don't think it's right that they stop giving childcare when a child turns 13. Who says that a 13-year-old doesn't need supervision? They need more. You can't leave a 13-year old to care for all the children. Without food stamps, I don't know what I would do. When there is no more public assistance, I don't know where I'll be. My main problem is the math. I go to school every other week and can't pass the math. The jobs want you to have math and reading. You don't get the job if someone is up here and you are down there.*

Ms. Carlton: *I enjoy working with the elderly. I have been looking all over for a job in a nursing home. Right now I am doing free labor. Why should they give us jobs when we do free labor? I want a job with benefits. Getting a home-health aid position doesn't have benefits. Some agencies have partial benefits and then you have to pay the rest. We want benefits but there are no jobs.*

I have not sat at home for two years. I come to work everyday. I have seven children. Welfare gives me $300 for food stamps that feeds my kids. I've got seven kids, and now they're changing the hours. We'll have to work until 5, and we get no vacation. We're working for the check. And then there is no time to study for math. You need time to learn this stuff, and once you get home it is too late.

Ms. Davis: *I was working as an aide and then I became ill. I had surgery and it took a long time to recover. I lost my job and have been in the circle for three years. I applied to St. James when I worked there, and they told me they had nothing. I worked in the laundry there, make beds at the nursing home. I have skills and can't get a job since my sickness.*

Ms. Ednes: [She is silent. When in agreement with a speaker, she would nod].

Ms. Fuller: *I just passed the GED, and I plan to find a job.*

At moments there were exploratory interchanges among the volunteers. Ms. Ednes wanted to know why Ms. Adams did not have a job, since she looked so well dressed and had a professional demeanor. Others questioned Ms. Barkley about the childcare arrangements she had put into place. There was an underlying tone of wanting recognition in regards to their testimony. I asked, *"What will make the program better?" "Kill the president."* (Everyone laughs.) I said, *"Well who would you put in his place?"* There is no answer, instead, *"I'd kill the mayor."*

I feel rage in the room. The target seems to be male leaders, and I think how surprised the volunteers would be if they knew how many female legislators supported welfare reform (Mink, 1998). What stands out for me is that the volunteers do not answer the question in the way I would expect, such as increased class time, reduced working hours, or provided job counseling. Instead, the response is to get rid of the male leader whom they perceive has caused misery and uncertainty in their lives.

Reflecting on the testimony of this second meeting, I realize that I heard the volunteers responding to the structural problem of feeling disempowered in accessing their human rights for economic security and educational opportunity. Emotionally, I sensed the volunteers' felt frustration and a threat of being unable to meet the basic human needs of food security, and environmental safety for their children (Galtung, 1994; Hershkoff & Loffredo, 1997; Roosevelt, 2001).

Two Interested Volunteers

From this second meeting, only Ms. Barkley (Esther) and Ms. Carleton (Betty) wanted to speak with me about participating in the study. Ms. Fuller (Agnes), who now for the second time avoided eye contact, had walked out. The others—Ms Adams, Ms. Ednes, and Ms. Davis—never made contact again regarding the study.

SETTING UP AN APPOINTMENT: THE LITERACY ISSUE

Esther and Betty announced that they would talk with me, but they did not want me to call them at home nor did they want to meet outside of the facility. They both asked, *"What's wrong with right here?"* When I asked Esther to write her name and department assignment on my pad, she wrote her name and then asked, *"Can you write activities?"* which I did. Betty refused to write anything. She just told me to find her when I came back.

At the time, I was not sensitive enough to the possibility that the volunteers might have problems with writing information. I was to learn that literacy was an obstacle that brought up shame, embarrassment, and frustration.

Betty found her way to avoid showing me her problem directly by coming up with a way for me to make contact with her, while Esther was willing to ask for help in writing a word she did not know how to spell.

Priority of Children Over Work

It took almost six weeks before I felt comfortable having another meeting. Betty and Esther wanted to talk with me, but they avoided signing the consent form. At the time, I did not know why. During this period, I talked with Camilla and Dorothea, who suggested I talk with the volunteer coordinator from the mandated program who worked in the third-floor dayroom. He was the only male volunteer in the program. I met with him after talking with Dorothea. He described the purpose of the program as providing an opportunity for the volunteers to get up in the morning and get to a workplace on time. He noticed that the mothers who had fewer than three children were more successful than those with three or more. When it came to choosing between the children or work, the children were always the first priority, making it hard for the women to find jobs. Oliker's (1995) study on work attachment of AFDC women in Wisconsin supports this notion of the volunteer coordinator, that when it came to protecting the lives of their children, work attachment behavior became secondary.

RESOLVING A FORMIDABLE RESISTANCE

I sensed the volunteers' formidable resistance to signing the consent form and that they would talk to me if they did not have to sign it. I did not know what to do. The feelings echoed at the last meeting made me feel pressured to do something for the volunteers. I went through a phase of developing proposal ideas for a reference library, a sisterhood committee, and a job readiness group. I questioned what kind of research I was doing and if it would be all right if I organized these activities for the volunteers, considering that my job was to conduct interviews. I was convinced that was never going to happen. The more despair I felt, the stronger the resistance became on the part of volunteers. Although none of this was voiced, it was still clear. Camilla said to just give it time, that "the girls" would get used to me and one day would just sign the form.

The problem was not only a trust issue. I did not understand that what the volunteers wanted and what I wanted were different. When they came to the meetings, they may have been hoping that someone was coming to take political action on their behalf to change their circumstances or to get them a job. I wanted to know their stories, but what would that do for them? It is possible that the volunteers felt let down by my purpose and that I could not meet their immediate needs for employment.

This conflict made me suffer, but it changed my own reserved perspective about hiding my feelings from the volunteers. As the weeks went by, I felt a closeness developing with the volunteers, but nothing was happening.

Gordimer's (1980) statement, "The resistance brought us closer although we didn't move" (p. 121) also describes how trust developed as I accepted the volunteers' resistance while still staying connected whenever personal contact was made. I managed my anxiety by talking with my husband Edward, exploring my own resistances in psychoanalysis, considering strategies with my support group, and communicating with my committee members who posed good questions and suggestions.

Fortified by my network of support, I was determined to call another recruitment meeting. Dorothea suggested that I organize the meeting myself. She felt the volunteers were getting used to me and would appreciate my asking them to participate in the meeting. Although I was apprehensive, I contacted the volunteers on the third floor. They didn't want any part of the study because they felt I was doing it only to get something for myself. Dolores, the head volunteer of the second-floor dayroom, encouraged volunteers on the second floor to come to the meeting.

THIRD MEETING WITH "THE GIRLS": PRIVACY ISSUES

On the day of the meeting, the room slowly filled up. I brought two boxes of doughnuts and placed them in the middle of the table. There were two rows filled with volunteers seated and several standing. Dolores sat directly across from me. There was silence. I noticed Betty, Esther, and Agnes sitting in the second row. It was the moment to start introducing myself.

Ellen: *I am going to be direct with you. Those of you who don't know me, my name is Ellen and I am a student. I am working on a dissertation project to learn about the experiences volunteers are having in being prepared for the workplace. I want you to know that I have talked about this project with Dorothea for over two years, and I have her support. I have worked here in the past and I wanted to do the project here.*

In order to do this project, I need your permission. When I first started the project, I was very nervous about it. I felt like

an intruder at first, and I can understand how you might have felt. Who is this person that wants to interview me?
   Now I have been here for two months. I no longer feel that way. I feel so certain the project is important. I know there are issues of trust. Why would you trust me? The types of questions I want to ask you are about your experiences here like, what kind of work do you want to do, what kind of training do you want, what do you enjoy the most? I do not want to intrude on your personal life.

In unison, the volunteer shook their heads in agreement. They seemed to resonate with my respecting their privacy.

Esther: *Betty and I have been talking to you and it's no big deal.*

The volunteers began to eat the doughnuts. The tension in the room loosened up. I confronted the problem of signing the consent forms. First, I describe what a consent form is and its protective purpose for the volunteer.

Ellen: *I want you to tell me right now, what harm can come to you if you give me permission?*
Dolores: (looks around the room and pauses) *There will be no harm. There is nothing wrong. It is okay. We will give you permission.*

Dolores then questioned me in detail about what the interviewing and consent process would entail. When I answered her questions satisfactorily, she communicated a look of acceptance to everyone in the room. Suddenly everyone was talking over each other. It was hard to listen to all the voices as they became stronger and louder. The concerns they raised touched upon the problem of unsupervised young teenagers caring for younger siblings in the late afternoon, when mothers were still at the worksite, and when unexpected events occur that the teenager cannot handle at home. For example, one little girl had died when she hit her head on the kitchen counter, and the older sibling panicked, unable to call his mother or anyone else for help. From the perspective of the volunteers, children die because of inadequate provisions for childcare and desperate attempts to comply with the mandated work program.
    Issues of unfairness were expressed regarding summer youth employed at the nursing home. Agnes asked everyone, *"How come they hire the summer youth and they can't hire us? It's not that the young shouldn't get jobs, but we're here, why can't they pay us?"* The need for recognition, honor, and respect turns to shame, embarrassment, and a sense of feeling

demeaned when the volunteers are told there will be "a breakfast for the volunteers." Betty describes how all the volunteers in the program had come to work that morning dressed up, but when they arrived for the breakfast, they were told the event was for "the church volunteers" and were sent back to their floor assignments. Esther states, *"We are never given credit or shown appreciation."*

Many of the volunteers joined in a discussion about the need for goal oriented training and education that would lead them to a job. Their experience showed them that skilled training is expensive and they would need scholarships. One volunteer asked, *"I want training to become a certified nursing assistant, but it costs $400. How can I pay that?"*

The underlying fear behind not getting the necessary training was that if they were not employable and could not find a job and their time limit was up, they would be in danger of losing their children to BCW (Bureau of Child Welfare). As one volunteer commented, *"BCW is going to take away our kids when we get thrown off the rolls and we have no jobs. More and more foster care programs are growing. They're getting ready to take away our children. It's already happening."*

This group of volunteers predicted that violence and crime in the community is the outcome of welfare reform. As one volunteer put it, *"When the benefits end in this community, there's going to be riots, stealing and killing. Your five dollars is my five dollars."* Holding this future at bay in the present was the existence of the "circle," a result of the non-event transition. Instead of making the transition to work, the volunteers repeated the workfare cycle over and over. While they are frustrated with feeling they are not getting closer to a job, there is some relief that they still have time.

In this third meeting comes a deeper discussion of the issues the volunteers face, such as the immediate attention required for the conditions of childcare for both young and older children. The mothers hold between themselves a system of attempting to manage work and family, with many adaptations that fail and cause suffering for all family members. When Connie spoke about this, she implied that the mothers in the program were making compromising decisions that could not be verbalized for fear of losing their children.

The Participants' Motivation: Change Society's Perceptions of Welfare Mothers

Six volunteers stepped forward to become participants in the research: Agnes, Betty, Dolores, Connie, Esther, and Florence. In preparatory discussions about the interview process, I asked them what they would like to get out of the study. A common theme among the volunteers was for the research to show their experiences in order to change society's negative perceptions of welfare mothers and to ensure the protection of children's well-being when benefits are terminated.

In this early stage, I gained a macro-view of what was on the minds of the volunteers. Economic and food security issues, educational opportunities, child protection, and the need for recognition and respect at the worksite were the initial concerns about which they wanted me to know.

doi:I0.1300/J004v23n03_04

Chapter 5

Promises to Keep:
Portraits of the Volunteers

SUMMARY. "Promises to keep" is a theme that weaves in and out of the experiences of the participants, from the past to the present. In this chapter, I present my impressions of the participants with this theme in mind. Demographic information is also integrated into the portraits. However, what I say about the participants comes from my subjective experience of spending many months in their presence. This chapter lays the groundwork for the stories of their experiences in their own words that are found in the subsequent chapters. doi:10.1300/J004v23n03_05 *[Article copies available for a fee from The Haworth Document Delivery Service: 1-800-HAWORTH. E-mail address: <docdelivery@haworthpress.com> Website: <http://www. HaworthPress.com> © 2007 by The Haworth Press, Inc. All rights reserved.]*

KEYWORDS. Portraits, job ready, maternal care

[Haworth co-indexing entry note]: "Promises to Keep: Portraits of the Volunteers." Greer, Ellen. Co-published simultaneously in *Occupational Therapy in Mental Health* (The Haworth Press, Inc.) Vol. 23, No. 3/4, 2007, pp. 57-70; and: *Women's Immersion in a Workfare Program: Emerging Challenges for Occupational Therapists* (Ellen Greer) The Haworth Press, 2007, pp. 57-70. Single or multiple copies of this article are available for a fee from The Haworth Document Delivery Service [1-800-HAWORTH, 9:00 a.m. - 5:00 p.m. (EST). E-mail address: docdelivery@haworthpress.com].

INTRODUCTION

In this chapter, I present the portraits of the six study participants: Dolores, Betty, Florence, Agnes, Connie, and Esther. Each had a life view driven by a promise made to herself in response to unique experiences of growing up with their mothers and grandmothers. Although each participant had a different promise, all promises were aimed toward their relationship with their children and were underpinned by their own standard of maternal care. The process of moving from welfare to the workfare program highlighted the past promises each woman had made to herself because she faced the challenge of becoming job ready and the stresses and strains that would place on her daily family life. The uncertain nature of the workfare program forced the participants to reflect on whether they would be able to keep their promise for their children.

DOLORES:
ALWAYS FOLLOW THE RULES:
ACT ON WHAT IS RIGHT

Dolores inspired cooperation. It was pure chemistry. Once in her presence, I was asking, "How can I help you with your activity?" With Dolores standing in the middle of the dayroom and delegating tasks to the volunteers, the room became organized and prepared for the residents within minutes. Other volunteers began to enter the back doorway and Dolores transported them in single file as they took their places in the room. Dolores was in charge. She was the head volunteer of the second-floor dayroom.

I met Dolores when she asked me to stand in front of Mrs. Stevens and model exercises to music. I became part of the line, Betty and Esther standing respectively to my left and right. With her crisp husky voice, like a breathy Peruvian flute ascending and descending quick passages, she enchanted all of us with her energy and imagination.

Her warm laughter, sense of justice, and responsibility was born out of pain, survival, and finding true love. Dolores was guided by rules: knowing what is right, identifying destructiveness, and acting to preserve goodness–even if it meant going underground. Learning about humane treatment began early in her life. As a six-year-old, newly emigrated from Santo Domingo, 14th of 15 children, she wanted to have the same freedom that the boys in her family had. Her teacher found her a disturbance in school and her mother could not control her. No one could handle Dolores. She found her way into the wards of Crestmore, a mental institution, somewhere around the ages of 8 to 10 years of age; she remained there the rest of her childhood. Becoming a keen observer and participant of institutional life, Dolores was sensitive to care-giving practices in any environment and responded to social injustices by taking actions for change.

Now 45, a mother of three children (ages 23, 18, and 10), grandmother of three (ages 10, 6, and 4), and living with her partner, 13 years her junior, Dolores created a new life for herself that began with the birth of her youngest son 10 years ago. Her life was devoted to creating an environment for her son to be nurtured. After Dolores was in the program for two years, she realized that *"Just being there for her son"* was not enough. She knew it was time to get an education, to nurture herself so that she could give to her child. School gave Dolores a new way to be with her family. Home life became structured around rules for study and play. The giant sunflower in her garden at home, along with the antenna planted in the soil to bring in energy from thunderstorms, are a metaphor for Dolores's relationship with learning and her family–she stands for energy, creation and growth.

She was the nursing home's guardian angel and when she left for another assignment, her friends missed her and the rhythm in the dayroom changed. In her new assignment, cooking in a shelter for homeless women, she has to stand on a chair to stir rice in huge tall pots that feed hundreds. She was given that assignment after she had threatened to report poor sanitation conditions in another part of the shelter. That is Dolores, always on the lookout to make things right.

Dolores's heartaches included her son John, who was incarcerated. They had been estranged for some time, but she wanted to contact him again. She dictated a letter to him that I wrote for her, which began her many visits with him that year. That summer, she said that her son was dying of cancer. He was in solitary confinement and she could petition his release, *"I know my son. If he comes home, he will be out there and I don't want to suffer for anyone he hurts. It will just happen."*

Dolores understood destructiveness. She had been abandoned by her mother, institutionalized, and later battered; then she crossed over to prostitution, drugging (using and selling), and incarceration. She encountered a near-death experience and then found herself slipping into an emotional breakdown. Yet she was in her home, overflowing with life and relationships. How did she survive such adversity?

Rutter (1987) points out that children with just one adult caring for them have more positive outcomes than those with no significant adult caring for them. Dolores was fortunate to have two people who loved her. At Crestmore, a nurse had wanted to adopt her, but when Dolores's mother refused to give up custody, Dolores ran away and lost this relationship. She almost died. Then she met the second person who loved her, and he did not let her go but nurtured her back to life. Her young husband set an example of doing the right thing in the way that he cared for her. Dolores internalized this caring experience, and it played a role in helping her to rebuild her life.

BETTY:
YOU CAN COUNT ON ME FOR STABILITY

Betty came to the second recruitment meeting; she was the woman with the sleeping child on her lap, whose trunk fell over the tabletop, breathing quietly as she slept on the hard surface. Esther, sitting to Betty's right, became her dearest friend and support. Betty was always at the worksite, even though she traveled a very long distance to be there. Coming to the nursing home was her *"bread and water,"* for if she did not take care of herself and her family, no one would.

Betty was a 38-year-old African-American mother of seven and was still coping with the sequalae of growing up as a child of intergenerational homelessness, neglect, and abuse. Her glowing high cheekbones, streetsmart twinkle in her eyes, and her cheerful presence disguised her sadness that she connected to the stresses of her life. The nursing home was Betty's dream. The environment contained much of what she needed: safety, structure, and an opportunity to care for others. In a voice of bewilderment, she expressed the anxious feelings of uncertainty: *"I don't know what will happen after this, don't know where I will go . . . This is the job I always wanted and now they're going to take this away from us. You can't get comfortable."*

Betty knew that she needed flexibility and a work setting that would tolerate her coming in late because of her children's medical appointments. The nursing home had accepted her best attempt to follow the rules because she was dependable and fit in.

She dressed neatly, in jeans or khaki pants with a bold plaid blouse or tee shirt and sneakers. A red cap covered her yellow curls, or a black stretch bandana tied in the back made her look like an adolescent. Some days she wore a sleek asymmetrical shining golden bob, shaping her beautiful face. She was confident, a woman who can stand on her own two feet. She did not think of the past. Underneath her confidence, Betty struggled with shame because of her marginal literacy. She had fears about her health, of being killed, and of being homeless again. She desperately wanted to escape from her older sons who were living chaotic and violent lives in her home. Talking about her older son's suicide attempt, Betty detailed how he shot himself, but without any emotion in her voice. Months later, she reported that one of the Bloods had cut into *"seven layers of his arm,"* as if it were a daily skirmish.

Guns, drugs, and gangs had been everyday experiences for Betty, having lived many years with her husband who had a drug territory in the neighborhood. Since his incarceration and deportation, Betty had to once again adjust to a life of poverty, while her adolescent children followed in their father's footsteps.

Betty's father had died of a drug overdose when she was small. Her drug-addicted mother had lived in the street, and her grandmother who raised her had been alcohol dependent. At the time of the interviews, Betty's mother had already died of AIDS, and her grandmother was in a nursing home. Betty and her siblings stayed close together and collaborated on ways to fill their empty stomachs. She and her sister made a promise, talking in the quiet of the night, that when they grew up, they would always be there for their children, who would never starve or be without lights or gas. Hence, Betty will do almost anything to prevent her children from experiencing hunger. If she ends up as she anticipates, without a job and homeless because there are no jobs for someone like her who cannot read or write well enough, she states she will beg on the trains. She would never consider selling her body, stealing, or accepting her sons' money from drug-related activities. What did Betty want from this research? *"When they cut people off don't cut off the children. They need to eat. Who's going to feed them?"* Talking with Betty changed me.

Her growing up in a life of poverty, drugs, violence, and no roots to count on overwhelmed me, and the telling of her story deeply upset me. It led me to read about the impact of psychosocial trauma that occurs in societies in armed conflict (Martin-Baro, 1994). I linked this to the urban war zone of Betty's past and present life. She was modest, yet she understood the impact her story had on me: *"I say I'm going to write a story about my life and then I say no, because I say if people read my book, they might cry."*

FLORENCE: SOMEONE WILL BE THERE FOR MY KIDS

I met Florence when I was sitting in the dayroom talking with Betty about training. As I gazed toward the back of the room, I noticed a woman in a white uniform walk confidently over to us, sit on the arm of Betty's chair, and join in the conversation. Florence did not work in the dayroom but was assigned to the nursing department to assist in care-giving activities. Volunteers assigned to nursing were given uniforms, so their status was disguised by the "whites" they wore each day. In contrast, the volunteers assigned to other departments wore casual clothes, usually jeans, blouse, and sneakers, that identified them as "the girls" or the welfare volunteers.

It was not clear that Florence was a volunteer until she expressed her frustration with the program, complaining that the workshops to help women get jobs were for women who had low self-esteem. Women like her needed more advanced training, she said, particularly the certification course that cost more than $100. Taking the course would help her meet the requirements to be a certified nurse's assistant. Her main focus was to get this additional training to ensure her employability. The only problem was obtaining the money to pay for the course.

A 38-year-old single mother of three young children under 10 years of age, Florence appeared determined to achieve an employed status. She had been raised in England by her Caribbean mother who had trained as a nurse there. At age 12, Florence, her mother, and her siblings immigrated to this country after her father had abandoned his family, leaving them homeless. Florence's maternal aunts were both nurses in the United States and had the means to help stabilize the family in a new country. In her adolescence, Florence found it difficult to adjust to her new inner-city culture. While her mother attended college late at night to gain her advanced certification in nursing, Florence floundered and then dropped out of school. Aspects of this acculturation experience had a profound effect on Florence.

She promised herself that when she had children and if she worked or she to college at night, there would always be someone there for her children. Having an unsupervised experience as an adolescent led her to believe that trouble for the child begins in that moment.

Pregnancy came late to Florence, and thankful for her three children, she chose a medical procedure to prevent the future conception of children. The father of her children was living in a Caribbean country, and Florence was prepared to raise her children alone. She had learned early on that she could only rely on herself and the support of her family.

Her notion of how much she could accomplish as a single mother of three children was realistic. Although some family members were against her wanting to become a certified nurse's assistant, she felt she needed to pace herself in building a career: *"I have to go slow, one step at a time. That's the way for me."* She took *"being looked down upon"* by her sister in stride. There was family pressure for children to become doctors, lawyers, or nurses, but Florence was not going to let that stand in her way.

During the first and second interviews, Florence described her workfare experience in glowing terms. She was hopeful that the skills she was learning from her workfare assignments in the hospital and now at the nursing home would prepare her for a job with benefits. She felt reassured that she would have excellent recommendations and that her skills would be in demand. She only needed money to take the test.

Imperceptibly Florence communicated a disjunction in her feelings about all the new rules of the workfare program. Although she would say, *"Oh, working in the program until 5:00 pm is no problem, "* several minutes later she would express her discomfort about having to have someone take care of her children every day after school. The desire to be self-sufficient and to be a provider for her children was strong, yet underneath Florence yearned to be home with them after school.

After a year went by, great excitement in the nursing home arose; Florence had left in the winter and the rumor was that she was working. The news inspired many volunteers eager to know that it was possible to find work after a workfare assignment. One day, a volunteer in contact with Florence reported that Florence was struggling financially and did not have a job. The system had made an error and had thrown her off the system. She was home, without an assignment and without the money to pay her bills.

What really happened? Getting back into the system takes time. Florence was waiting for a new workfare assignment that she found acceptable. In the meantime, she could not pay her bills and had no financial resources to pay for the certified nurse's assistant course that had been her focus the year before. In between, she had been offered a private case to care for a man with a terminal illness. The case lasted two weeks. Even though she had to travel four hours a day, she wished she still had the work. On the other hand, she admitted that while all of this waiting was difficult, she knew good would come of it and she was glad to be home with her children during this break.

AGNES: LOOK AFTER YOURS FIRST

Agnes was like a woman warrior. Instead of graceful clothes and gold jewelry, she wore a mean-guarded countenance reminiscent of aged silver armor that has lost its luster. Understanding the meaning of her look gets a person past it. The hidden softness underneath can shock one to tears. That is how I felt after she attended three of my recruitment meetings, each time gazing away or looking through me–until the last time, when I spoke with emotion and stood up at the end of my talk, she was two inches away from me and quietly said with a smile, *"I'll do it for you."* This did not mean we were friends. She kept her distance from me and the other volunteers. She was a volunteer assigned to the second floor dayroom program.

In contrast to the other volunteers, she most often looked serious and avoided joking around with anyone. Her attention was usually focused on her agitated patient, Alice, who seemed only to be calmed by Agnes's presence.

A 33-year-old African-American single mother of three daughters, Agnes had been in the program for two years. The past year, she had succeeded in obtaining her GED, and for a woman who keeps practically everything under wraps in the work setting, she flaunted this achievement like a precious dagger before the other volunteers. She appeared willing to draw blood and fight. Agnes's stories wove in and out: her life, her children, her hurt, her daughter's sexual abuse, her rage at her brother, her daughters' behavior in school, her behavior when she was their age, not wanting to abuse them, and, finally, her abuse: *"There wasn't no child abuse in those days,"* meaning that when she was a child, a parent could beat a child; there was no legal protection.

She only spoke intermittently about the workfare program, and her short stories about the program were like rests in a musical composition. They would accentuate the phrases that came before and after. Talk about the program was followed by thoughts about her relationship with the father of her children, her ex-husband, and this pattern continued throughout the interviews.

She was now responsible for her family. Raising a family and living together for 17 years, she decided to go on welfare in case her husband would leave her. And he did. And she protected herself as best she could through gaining basic resources from public assistance. In the mid-1990s, she lost her father, then she lost her three-day-old infant son, and then her husband left. Agnes did not talk about pain, hate, or love, but her anger was as livid as hot melted glass. It came through in her language–words and phrases such as *scratch, pluck, knock the shit out of him, turn on her,* and *smack*–yet she showed caring actions with the nursing home residents and hyper-vigilance with her three daughters: *"I don't hit mines, and no one hits mines."*

Agnes noticed that her interest in helping others became stronger since the time of her father's illness, then caring for the elderly in the nursing home, and now her mother's need for her attention since her challenge with hemiplegia from a recent stroke. Agnes was interested in pursuing training to become a certified home health aid, but she was concerned that the workfare program would not approve the time or expense.

After three months, Agnes was stressed with multiple problems. She was spending more time with her mother to help manage her diabetic condition that was out of control, she herself was recovering from surgery, and her daughters were acting out in school. So many problems in caring for others changed Agnes's mind about becoming a home health aid, and she decided to train in engineering and construction instead. She reported feeling too depressed, that getting close to the patients with whom she worked and then losing them was too much for her to handle.

In the second interview, Agnes briefly uttered the word *college* but leaves it in the air because her first goal is to get a job. She worried that training for a job with a utility company to read meters would be too boring. She pushed this aside and then talked about how she managed her daughters–tight control but not as tightly as she had been controlled: "*I am just beginning to express my feelings about how I was raised by my mother and father.*" While she never talked about the poverty with which she lived, she did describe the stigma of being poor as a child: "*I was one of nine. My mother didn't have anything to give us, and they used to point, 'Look at her hair, sneakers she got on.' They did that and I just walked away from them.*" Her childhood experience gave her the sense of what a good mother must do, and from this personal knowledge she developed a set of rules to follow:

> "*Look after yours first. You have to take care of yourself. Make sure that they have. Not like some mothers who only wear nice clothes and jewelry. But the baby looks like a bum, like they haven't combed their hair in a week. Mine gets their hair every Sunday.*"

Agnes was a vigilant mother stressed by her constant worry for the safety for her daughters, and while she wanted to get off public assistance and work, she also resented the "*quality time the program is taking from mothers and fathers from their children.*"

CONNIE:
I WILL SHOW MY CHILDREN HOW TO BEAT FEAR

Connie, a vivacious 28-year-old Panamanian-born woman, mother of three children (ages, 3, 7 and 10), had been a volunteer at the nursing home for over a year. Connie's voice and actions were fast, sharp and emotional, underpinned with a smoky anger fused with a kindness and moral responsibility. These qualities of goodness were shaped by her maternal grandmother's words, which were offered to soften the blows of a harsh experience through which Connie had to live. Her grandmother's words serve as her source of rules for living life:

My grandmother, now that is a woman that I can tell you. You can learn a lot from her. I lost her in '95. All she told me on her dying bed was "What I taught you try and use it." And I try to do that. She told me the rule of life. If someone does something for you, you always be grateful. Help people. And even if you have a problem, there is always tomorrow. She said to me, "Always remember to give your kids what you never had. Don't let a bad situation make your heart burst from there. And don't ever give people that experience."

When Connie was seven, her mother became ill and her grandmother stepped in and raised Connie and her brother. Connie had a bad relationship with her mother growing up and did not understand her mother until after her grandmother died. She thought her past as harsh and unbearable. When Connie was an adolescent, her grandmother convinced her to tell her mother that she was five months pregnant. This set the stage for years of turmoil, for her mother forced her to have an abortion:

The worst experience I had was losing that child. That drove me crazy. That is why I didn't finish school. I couldn't go to school. I was a junior and it messed me up completely. I used to hear a baby crying and I would say, "Is that mine?" Maybe that is why I am punished because I cannot have no girls. Maybe it was a girl. That is what haunts me now and then, not all the time.

Connie was married and had three sons. Several years ago, her husband, a drug dealer, was incarcerated over a drug war dispute. Connie had been raising the children on her own with help from her mother, mother-in-law, and brother. Her oldest son missed his father and had trouble adjusting to life without him. Her seven-year-old was disabled with Erbs Palsy, and Connie was teaching him to overcome his fear of his new prosthetic arm. Her youngest child seemed to make the least demands on Connie, for he rarely emerged as an interview topic.

Connie's children were her motivation. She dreamed that they would be proud of her, that they would say, *"My mommy is working. She got off the welfare system and bounced back."* Bouncing back had been a journey of self-discovery for Connie, and it was during her workfare assignment in the nursing home that she had to face her nasty attitudes, her not caring at the beginning, and her depression in response to being forced to be there every day or to be terminated from the system.

Over the course of a year, Connie learned to care about the patients. She also bonded with her peers, whom she said were *"in the same shoe"* as she, and she discovered that working as a team forges a space of attention where friendships become the catalyst for change.

Her most critical challenge was coping with her marginalized status as a welfare volunteer under the supervision of a professional middle-class Hispanic woman, Camilla. She was determined to change and to work on her character and her relationship with her supervisor. Connie saw patterns and stages in all she did. She was always learning or teaching her mother, her brother, her sons, the new volunteers at orientation, or her peers at the nursing home.

After more than a year had passed, Connie reflected on her experience and offered some advice for others who start the mandated work program:

> *You got to pass through fear. You got to pass through wondering. You got to pass through "Am I going to be able to do it?" You've got to pass through four things. Okay, orientation is a whole. You got to learn what the program is about, what it is offering you, what you are going to do about it, and how you're going to get off the system. You might not like it, but you got to deal with it.*

ESTHER:
YOU'VE GOT TO BE THERE

Esther stood out when I met the volunteers at a recruitment meeting. She appeared dignified with her nicely-tailored Kelly-green pantsuit and her precisely straight and styled hair. Her voice was stronger than her peers as she articulated the injustices and frustrations of workfare. Her concerns were centered on the need for supervision of teenage children. She explained how, from her perspective, the TANF program was inequitable in providing financial resources for teens over 13, leaving them without supervision if a mother could not pay the babysitter for an extra child.

Esther was in a successful place in her life. She had completed a drug rehabilitation program and had remained clean for six years. Concurrent with beginning the workfare program, she was given custody of her three children and one nephew whose mother was drug dependent. Her commitment was focused on being there for her children, helping her nephew, and getting an education. She idealized work. She did not believe anyone would hire her without a GED, although she did have seasonal employment at an amusement park.

Her openness about her lack of basic literacy skills and her honesty about the pointlessness of the program made me want to help her. One day when she expressed her being worried about her difficulty learning multiplication and division, I asked her if she had ever used flashcards for practice. She did not know what flashcards were, so I brought in a set in for her. Esther learned math quickly, and by the end of the year, she was helping her own children with reading and math.

What amazed me most about Esther was her appreciation for the supportive relationships she had had with women throughout her life, particularly during the time when she had lost her children to other mothers. Her sister had cared for three of her sons, and her baby had been given to a foster mother. Both women had made sure that Esther had contact with her children while she was in recovery, encouraged her to get on her feet, and retained a relationship with the children after Esther had taken them back.

Esther's compassion and understanding for the foster mother who grew to love her child is striking.

> *They were out of my life when they were young. My youngest son was two weeks old. The other ones were bigger, but they weren't too far behind. The baby was two weeks, the other was one, and the other was four or five. Now the only one getting to know me is the baby. See, the others stayed at my sister's house. I came in and said, "Hi ya," and stuff like that, but with my three, the baby was the one who had to get to know me.*
>
> *The reason I got to know him was the foster mother who used to bring him and write little notes to me, telling me to get my life together. She could never take the place of being his mother, because she is Puerto Rican. She sees him because she is his godmother. She helped me out a lot in the program to keep myself together and keep the kids and stuff. She'd bring my son to see me all the time. I am his mother now.*

Esther explained how difficult it was to take her child away from the foster mother because she had been quite aware of their attachment to each other.

> *He came home and it was hard for her. I took him just out of her life like that. I could tell every time we got to talking and she knew he was going to leave, the tears in her eyes. I always told her, "You ain't going to miss him. We are both going to have him," so I take him to her all the time. . . . He knows that whenever he wants to see her I take him over . . . I take him to Manhattan 'cause he goes for the weekends. He's bonded. He knows I'm his momma. I guess that*

is how she taught him. Like she told me, she could never take the place of his mother.

Esther's story of her cooperative relationship with the foster mother describes her respect of relationships in general. She takes others' feeling into account and expects to be treated in the same way. Her peers in the nursing home recognized this quality about her; she formed close attachments with Betty, Dolores, and Connie–all three cooperate well when working together in the dayroom.

What did Esther want out of her life now that she was starting over? .

What I want out of life is a nice job. I want to be able to take care of my kids and not worry about this PEP thing [program]. I want school and stuff. You can't get no good job if you don't know how to read.

REFLECTIONS

The participants were able to mold an individual promise from the pain they had experienced from their past loss, abandonment, hunger, abuse, and yearning for love–a promise that each carried with her over many turbulent years. Their promises seemed to be a means for surviving their pain and offered a particular kind of motivation to attempt to do better for their children. The nature of the participants' promises fit into particular life-affirming categories, underpinned by moral actions, values, and an ethic of care that help explain each participant's struggle and strategy for survival.

Dolores's promise was to preserve goodness. Having experienced the dark side of humanity, Dolores refused to succumb. She applied her understanding of destructive actions to many levels of human interaction, doing whatever she could to turn a bad situation into a good one. She constantly worked hard to communicate her values for humane treatment and education with those with whom she worked, as well as with her family.

Both Betty and Florence promised responsibility to their children. Having experienced abandonment and neglect by a parent and later inconsistent parental supervision instilled in both women a need to establish a caring and safe life for their children. Managing this promise required continuous planning and strategizing to ensure consistent food and shelter for their families.

Agnes promised vigilance. Closely monitored as a young girl, Agnes had learned about the desire to break away from family control. When she finally escaped the daily control of her family, she was forced to face her own inexperience. Acting on her anger at having been controlled, Agnes let things go, jeopardizing the life of her daughter. However, in response to her daughter's being sexually abused by her brother, Agnes reframed her concept of vigilance, and she promised she would protect her daughters from outsiders who could hurt them. This required her to keep her children's thoughts, feelings, and behaviors at the forefront and kept her on a constant alert for danger.

Connie promised to help others. Her promise to her grandmother that she would help others and not cause them pain taught her that through teaching and loving actions, she could help herself and her family. Actualizing this promise became part of Connie's daily interaction with others both at work and at home. By always asking herself, "What can I do to help this person," Connie connected with others, which, in turn, helped her to reformulate her aspirations for her future with her family.

Esther's promise was to be there for her children. Losing her children because of her drug addiction and incarceration provided her with an opportunity to discover the importance of maternal care and her need for her children. Her promise motivated her to rebuild her life with fierce determination, while at the same time honoring the help she received from other mothers throughout her journey to regain her maternal rights.

doi:10.1300/J004v23n03_05

Chapter 6

Surviving Adversity

SUMMARY. In this chapter, I present the theme "surviving adversity." While coding the transcripts of the volunteers' stories, two subthemes of surviving adversity emerged that were common in all the participants' stories: family disruption and lack of external controls in the environment. The stories reflect the strategies that may be developed to face life-threatening adversity. I first discuss the components of each subtheme and present a participant's story to highlight those components. doi:10.1300/J004v23n03_06 *[Article copies available for a fee from The Haworth Document Delivery Service: 1-800-HAWORTH. E-mail address: <docdelivery@haworthpress.com> Website: <http://www.HaworthPress.com> © 2007 by The Haworth Press, Inc. All rights reserved.]*

KEYWORDS. Adversity, survival, family disruption, risk factors, protective factors

[Haworth co-indexing entry note]: "Surviving Adversity." Greer, Ellen. Co-published simultaneously in *Occupational Therapy in Mental Health* (The Haworth Press, Inc.) Vol. 23, No. 3/4, 2007, pp. 71-85; and: *Women's Immersion in a Workfare Program: Emerging Challenges for Occupational Therapists* (Ellen Greer) The Haworth Press, 2007, pp. 71-85. Single or multiple copies of this article are available for a fee from The Haworth Document Delivery Service [1-800-HAWORTH, 9:00 a.m. - 5:00 p.m. (EST). E-mail address: docdelivery@haworthpress.com].

Available online at http://otmh.haworthpress.com
© 2007 by The Haworth Press, Inc. All rights reserved.
doi:10.1300/J004v23n03_06

INTRODUCTION

Sometimes when I asked a simple question or when I was just listening, I would catch myself holding my breath as the volunteers' stories delicately stepped from the present into the past. It was as if I were standing on a stone in a pond and, with an unconscious slip, found myself with both feet in the water. In the splash of contact with the elements of a life history, a story is told, linking the past with the present. Bal, Crew, and Spitzer (1999) call stories of recall "cultural memories," signifying memory as a cultural, as well as individual or social, phenomenon. They consider a cultural memory as something performed, although not necessarily consciously or willfully, an "activity occurring in the present, which the past is continuously modified and redescribed even as it continues to shape the future" (p. vii). As the researcher, I assumed an unexpected sense of responsibility. It was difficult to integrate the volunteer's harsh childhood experiences, and I was overcome with wanting to do something about it. Their stories of the past were told with poignant emotion in the present, as if the past were still alive and I was witnessing their adversity. The stories of their histories were a link to their problems of their present and seemed to shape their attitudes and behavior in the hope that such adversity would not be repeated. It seemed as if understanding the past would help determine what needs had to be addressed in the present for success in the future.

Martin-Baro (1994) reminds us, "Any human community must concern itself with the survival of its members." To help others survive, we need to know the obstacles that are in their way. As a researcher, my contribution is to tell what I learned through the participants' voices as they told their stories in their own words.

Family Disruption

Reasons for family disruption during childhood varied among the participants. Betty's mother had been drug-addicted and handed over her caregiver role to the maternal grandmother, who lacked the emotional and material resources to care for Betty and her siblings. Dolores's family was disrupted when her mother left her father behind in their homeland. Later, Dolores was torn from her family when she was adjudicated to live in a state hospital. Connie's mother had suffered from an undisclosed illness, and Connie's care was given over to her maternal grandmother. Florence's father had jeopardized the lives of his family when he no longer paid the mortgage on their home in England, leaving Florence, her mother, and her siblings homeless. Emigrating eventually to the United

States had been a culture shock for Florence, and she had great difficulty adjusting. Esther's mother had been a substance user who provided inconsistent care, although she tried to manage drinking and motherwork. Her father had been incarcerated several times and never returned home to his family. While Agnes had the most stable family life living with two working parents, they had been challenged by great poverty and lacked necessary resources.

Listening to the stories and frequently rereading the transcripts, I realized that the participants were telling me the different ways they had survived. Survival in their early years was usually attributed to a maternal or sisterly figure, legitimate and illegitimate activities, and an ethic of care in taking responsibility for younger siblings or their own newborns as young teen mothers. Betty's story touches upon some of these strategies for survival.

BETTY

Betty's mother had been a young woman when she arrived in the East in the early 1960s from a town in the South. Betty did not know much about her parents' background; in fact, the only thing she knew about her father was that he had died from drug use. After he died, Betty's mother, also a drug user, could no longer care for her children and took up residence on the streets. Betty's maternal grandmother became the children's primary caregiver. Betty's voice was often filled with sarcasm when she spoke of her grandmother: *"She really didn't raise us. We just stayed with her. She drank, too, so it was like we just there."* Betty and her siblings witnessed a total family collapse when Betty's mother moved into the streets:

> *I used to pray all the time that my mother would stop using drugs and stuff. I used to pray for my little brother when my mother had him, 'cause she used to sleep with him in the car. And I used to pray that I see him. And when I get a little money baby-sitting and stuff like that I buy a little outfit for him. When he come, I could take him 'cause I was young you know. And is why like I said I didn't finish school.*

At a young age, Betty became a caregiver, dropping out of school to care for her younger siblings to prevent their removal from the family.

The children had been either living on the streets with her mother or unsupervised in the grandmother's home:

> *I took care of them. I didn't want to see them in the street taken away, so I used to wash all their clothes by hand and keep their hair combed. One of my sisters had eczema, had it real bad and used to stay in and out of the hospital, 'cause I was not able, but I took her anyway right. Sometimes they said I was too young, so they had to call somebody to give her a shot or something. I was underage. I used to take them to school and do their hair. Make sure they look nice and clean for school. I used to baby-sit them and come back and go shopping to buy them something. Now they big. They okay. One of them is in jail, but they still nice.*

Although Betty did her best to take care of the younger siblings, she struggled with physical hunger and cold:

> *I came up rough, the hard way. I have always been in and out of shelters. I know what it is like. I know what it's like not to have a plate of food on the table. I know what it is like not to have shoes on your feet. I know all about that.*
> *My grandmother used the cooking grease to comb my hair. She did the best that she can because my mother wasn't there, so she tried. She got welfare after a while. My grandmother was drinking, so the money used to go 'cause back then the checks were coming every 1st and 16th of the month. The next day, she would wake up and the money was gone because she was drunk. We were lucky. We ate that day, I am telling you! Sometimes we don't have gas for a whole year. We used to buy sternos. So I know what it is like not having the gas or light. There were days when you don't have food for three days. My grandmother would pick us up and put us in the bathtub. Another thing, the house was cold. If you didn't eat in three or four days, you be so homely you have to be picked up (laughing), to keep our feet warm, 'cause we were cold and we didn't have food.*
> *We used to look for bottles to get cookies and stuff 20 blocks a day. Looking for bottles, to eat, you know, cash them in. In the store, cash your bottle there. After a while they stopped, but you can do it now again. Yeah, cash in the bottles and buy a cookie. Cash in more and buy package of cookies for food, yeah. My brother used to do the stealing.*

He used to steal out of the meters where you put the quarters.
He would break the was alive. She was still in Manhattan and my
uncles were in Manhattan, too. They had money but we didn't have
no food. But you know, we made it through. The part I didn't like
was being weak all the time. You couldn't get sick. There was noth-
ing to get sick off of. How you going to get sick if you have not
strength? You can't get sick if you have no food in your stomach.
Sure wasn't the food that was poisoning us (laughing). So she didn't
have to worry about toilet tissue. You know, if she got some
change, she would buy some mush. She would mix up oatmeal into
a pot and mix it up for us. It was lumpy but it would stick to your
stomach. I raised off milk and juice and all that stuff.

When Betty's grandmother began to receive food from welfare, such
as cheeses, milk, and juice, she implemented a daily meal schedule to feed
the family. Regular staples brought 15 family members living together in
the grandmother's two-bedroom apartment.

We all got fed at the same time, but if you were not there you don't
eat. It can't be like no leftovers. There was 15 of us in one apart-
ment. It was two meals a day. It was breakfast, whenever it was,
and dinner. So everybody eat off of that. If we don't have welfare
food, then she would go to the store. It was cheap. You could buy
five pounds of chicken backs and cook that up with rice.

Holidays were especially difficult for Betty. There were no celebrations
in her grandmother's home, and some years they relied on the church for
food or presents.

We never had a tree, so we never knew what Christmas is like. We
didn't wake up to a tree in the morning. We didn't get presents.
The church did give us presents, or we go there and they have a lit-
tle Christmas party. We woke up on Christmas morning and there
was nothing to eat. We went to church to give us something to eat,
but they don't. We had nothing to eat. That is why I'm breaking my
neck to get for my kids. So they can never say they didn't get, I didn't
have it.

Betty's reaction to the neglect she experienced was to become a young
caregiver, while suffering the deprivations of her basic needs. She took on

the maternal role whenever possible and tried to survive hunger and cold in the absence of family protection.

Maternal or Sisterly Figure Connection

Of all the participants, Betty did not develop a strong relationship with a maternal or sisterly figure. She assumed a maternal role and helped the siblings survive by caring for their basic needs. Later, she helped her mother with food stamps when she had her own first child and received public assistance. Betty called herself *"the black sheep"* in the family. Although she had received love from the siblings for whom she had provided her best ministrations of care, she still believed there was no one to love her and no one to pimp her, that she had grown-up without affection.

Legitimate and Illegitimate Activities

Betty's activities for survival were interwoven with care for others and for herself. She baby-sat for money from an early age. She developed caregiving skills when responsible for caring for young children, and the money she earned she used to purchase "an outfit" for her younger sibling. Those caregiving activities for her siblings, such as dressing, combing hair, and taking care of medical needs, also enhanced her feelings of connection to them. When they went hungry, the siblings decided to sell bottles for cookies, and Betty and her siblings agreed that the brother would commit a crime (breaking into parking meters) to get money for food. They were left to their own devices, and most of the activities that Betty reported were legitimate and constructive in ensuring their survival. For example, in the later years when her grandmother received welfare food supplies, Betty learned that the successful activity of obtaining nourishment meant that she had to be at home at the right time or else no food would be available. With the new resource of daily meals came a structure that did not exist when the children had to strategize to find food. During her early adolescent years, welfare became a necessary means of survival in Betty's eyes.

CARE ETHIC

Instilled in Betty at a very young age was a desire to keep the family of children together. She worked very hard to provide a caring relation to her siblings and later on to her mother when she was dying of AIDS. Woven into her care ethic was a relationship with a higher power through prayer. She did not talk in detail about her relationship with God. However, when I think about how Betty developed a strong sense of responsibility to care for others in the face of everyday hunger and cold, I imagine she may have received inspiration and comfort from her spiritual life.

Lack of External Controls in the Environment

The subtheme of survival of the lack of external controls in the environment consisted of two components: risk factors and protective factors. Each component is discussed below.

RISK FACTORS

Several volunteers talked about "doing things I wasn't supposed to do" as adolescents. They were referring to behaviors that made them at risk for illiteracy, addiction, teen pregnancy, sexual and physical abuse, and, later, incarceration. The major types of risk factors emerging from the data were dropping out of school, dangerous relationships with men, drug addiction, teen pregnancy, trauma, and keeping experiences of abuse secret.

Without external controls in the contexts of the environments in which they lived, participants grew up without family protection. Betty had run from one home to another, dropped out of school, experimented with drugs, and became a victim of abuse of the male relatives living in her grandmother's home, as well as her mother's new husband. Dolores had run from the state hospital when her mother refused a nurse's request to adopt Dolores. This led to a journey searching for safety but only finding abuse, violence, and pregnancy. Esther had not gone to school, and her sister introduced her to a crack habit. Connie had become pregnant while living away from her parents. When her parents learned of her condition, they insisted on an abortion. In her rage at being forced to do this, she dropped out of school and became pregnant again. While Florence's mother attended college and worked, Florence was left to her own devices and eventually stopped going to school. Agnes, who had the most supervision of all the participants, was suddenly "let loose" at 17, when her mother felt she could no longer keep her from going out. Once the controls were lifted, Agnes became pregnant, drank, smoked, and was very carefree with her young child. Several years later, she discovered that her older brother had molested her daughter when Agnes was not watching carefully.

PROTECTIVE FACTORS

Against the harsh realities of adolescence, the participants also demonstrated protective behaviors to find support, either from a mother or grandmother, older siblings and friends, strangers who could provide refuge, public assistance to assuage hunger and provide shelter, or professional support from a therapist to heal the trauma of sexual abuse.

Gaining support from her mother and grandmother were essential for Connie's successful second pregnancy. Her father had been enraged. He envisioned his daughter as a *"crystal ball broken into 100 pieces. I am not going to put her back together again. She cannot live here."* However, Connie's mother fearlessly stood up to her husband, finding Connie shelter and supporting her throughout the pregnancy.

Florence had counted on the support of her older sister and friends during her high school years. Coming from England at age 12, Florence had had a difficult time assimilating into her new urban neighborhood. She entered the school system as a junior high school student and was placed in the gifted class. While Florence was in junior high, her mother worked as a nurse and was home at the end of the school day, but when Florence entered high school, her mother returned to college to earn credentials for her nursing position. Florence found her mother's absence after school hours and during evening hours intolerable.

> *My mother went back to college. I never really gave my mother a lot of trouble, but I never finished school and education was her number one thing. She went to college when I was 16. We were left to do whatever we wanted to do. Now a teenager with no supervision you know, I wasn't doing anything bad, but I didn't go to school. What it was, I had friends older than me. The school had two sessions. My sister was in the older grade. She went to school in the morning. I was with the ninth and tenth graders, and we went to school in the afternoon. Everything was going on when I should have been in school. A little was going on here, and my sister was able to go because she was out of school and I wasn't. I used to have to play hooky to hang out with them. That's why I was cutting class. I would sometimes end up in places that I should not have ended up in, but I never had friends that disrespected me.*
>
> *One thing I could say is that I had friends who looked after me. I had guys as friends who would talk to me and treat me as their sister. I just didn't want to go to school. School was too fast for me. The pace was too fast. Like here you learn something in a week*

*and they give you a test. I wasn't used to that. I really didn't like
school. When my mother was in college, we did what we wanted io
do. I learned from that. I want the father. If I have to work in the
evening, he has to work in the day so that someone is home to keep
an eye. I did things that my parents would have expected better.*

Esther talked about a similar feeling of not doing what she was supposed to do. She said her life growing up *"was terrible. I don't remember.
I couldn't have had too much of a good life because my mother used to
party, drink a lot of stuff."* On the other hand, Esther noted that her mother
was a good sewer: *"My mother was a good sewer. She made our clothes.
Being that I was in the house all the time, I used to make things. I didn't
want to hang out until I was older."*

Middle adolescence for Esther was noted for its behavior problems.
While her mother sent her to school each day, she had no idea whether that
was her daughter's destination.

*I did things I wasn't supposed to do. I barely went to school. I was
running around the streets, you know, hanging out and stuff. I could
have learned, I could have went to school. My mother sent us out to
go to school. My mother didn't let any of us stay in the house. We
were all sent out to go to school. I chose not to. I was in the tenth
grade, like a problem child myself. They put me in an all girls' school.
You know, I can't remember back that far, why I was like that, you
know. We were just there because we were bad. If you learned, you
learned, and if you didn't want to learn, they weren't forcing you.*

In a conversation, Esther and Betty compare their school experiences
and introduction into drugs.

Esther: *I was selling it and started doing it. You know, when you have
a lot of money and somebody tell you to try it, and right now in
the day, my baby sister got me to try it. She's still on it. She
introduce me to it. My younger sister and she still on it, and I
got her younger son now. She the one that introduce me. I didn't
know none. I was mostly babysitting and stuff like that now.*

Betty: *I did baby-sitting too.*

Esther: *That was like my thing.*

Betty: *My mother got worse and stuff like that, so I started staying
home smoking my little weed and stuff*

Esther: *And cutting out of school and stuff like that, you know. You
make that little money. I used to baby-sit and stuff like that.*

> *And then one day my sister said, "Try this." I tried it, and she used to catch me all the time and whine me for my money and never come back.*

Betty: *I never tried that.*

Esther: *I went to an outpatient program and I stopped. Before that, I got pregnant again, and I was doing it when I was pregnant. That's when they took my kids.*

Betty: *I was no angel. I was lucky when I took that second blow. It made me sick of dope, and I never tried it again. It was nice at first. My friend said, "Try it."*

Esther: *You were snorting?*

Betty: *Yeah, 'cause I know my mother was on drugs, and I didn't want to go that way, right? She said, "Come on. You know it ain't going to do nothing to you." And I said, "Are you sure?" And I took it. Understand I felt nice. (Esther and Betty laugh). A week later I went for another blow to two girls. I was sick like a dog. I was crawling on the floor. I said, "Lord, if you let me get better, I will not do it again."*

Esther: *I heard that gets you sick and everything. I know people that say it always gets you sick, so I was scared to try it. And when I tried that, crack took me down. The worst thing that happened to me was getting on those drugs.*

Betty and Esther had been trying to figure things out and managed to survive, although along the way, they both had their run in with the criminal courts because of drugs. Betty married a man who had a large drug territory and became involved in transporting drugs to get the money to pay for their home that was in foreclosure when her husband was incarcerated. Esther developed an expensive crack habit. She was incarcerated and then sent to a drug rehab facility.

DOLORES

Dolores's story reflects both subthemes of surviving adversity (family disruption and lack of external controls in the environment). In fact, family disruption, school failure, drugs, and running away led Dolores down what sociologist Esther Enos (2001) calls the path to prison.

In the 1950s, after World War II, when the United States was prospering and welfare was available to help immigrant families, a mother in her early thirties who had survived giving birth to 15 children (including four pairs of twins, two pairs of which survived) left her younger second husband in Santo Domingo and traveled with her brood of young children to New York City, the home of her two oldest children. Her next-to-youngest child (number 14), six-year-old Dolores, felt bewildered and confused. She wondered why they had they left their father behind and what they were doing "*in this new place.*" When Dolores talked about her first separation, leaving both her homeland and her father, she was still angry.

> *She never told us. I don't know why she never did because when she left my father, she did not explain nothing to us about coming to this country. All she said was, "Because I am no longer with your father, welfare is going to support us." She didn't explain why we were coming to this country. She left us blank.*

She learned from that experience that children can become disturbed by marital conflict. She was determined to communicate differently to her children.

> *You know, like my sons. I tell my sons when things happen. When me and his father get into an argument, he gets real nervous, and I tell my son, "Sometimes lovers react."*

Dolores often compares her life to that of her mother:

> *My mother was older than my father. He was young. So some of her kids were already married and had their own kids. See, like in my life, my husband is younger than me. My mother was like that.*

Dolores tried to understand her mother in telling her story. She was angry because she perceived that her mother had not been honest with her. She evaluated her mother's strengths and did not understand why a literate woman would lie to her children.

> *Why did mother lie to us so much? What sense did that make to lie to a kid? My mother knew how to read and write. I don't know why she never went to school. I just don't understand.*

Dolores reviews her mother's early history.

> *My mother was raised with her father and her mother abandoned her. Her father owned a store. My father didn't know how to read or write, so I guess we took after the father's side.*

Dolores wanted to assert that she was a spirited girl, in direct conflict with her mother's values. Dolores recalled that she started to act out when she began school in an urban neighborhood.

> *That is the only thing I remember or that is what I want to remember. They say you forget what you want to remember. She took me to school. And I had a problem with the teacher. I didn't realize what I was doing. But I was a bad girl though. I wanted to be a boy. I feel that they give boys more freedom. And because I was a girl, she didn't want to give me freedom. So, I act like a boy. I started fighting with boys, hitting my teacher. Everything boys do, so she couldn't handle me. They took me away from her, put me away in an institution. They said I made a lot of stories. I know it was a story. It was a teacher against a student. My mother said, "She's lying." So the judge said, if my mother said so, "She cannot be controlled."*

Dolores felt betrayed by her mother. Instead of fighting to keep her daughter, she supported the teacher's accusation. Once Dolores was institutionalized, her mother had minimal contact with her until a nurse at the facility wanted to adopt her. When Dolores's mother refused the nurse's request, Dolores ran away in anger. There did not appear to be any controls to prevent her from leaving the state hospital grounds. In the following excerpt, Dolores shared what precipitated her running away and the outcome of that experience.

> *The lady who wanted to adopt me took me downstate, down south, a lot of places. My mother never gave me, for adoption. They couldn't do that, but in the meantime she put me away and didn't see me for a couple of years. She didn't want to be bothered with me. So there was no room for the adoption. The lady signed the papers and everything.*

Her mother first attempted a reconciliation by writing a letter to Dolores.

> *All that time, my mother went back to court. My mother wrote me a letter which I didn't know how to read or write. Someone read it for me, and she told me, "Your mother said she was sorry. What you said about the teacher, the teacher did it to another kid, and the teacher got suspended, whatever." I didn't want to go back to her.*

She went back to court. They were going to put me up for adoption, but because she needed me to sign for adoption, they couldn't.

When the letter failed, Dolores's mother showed up at the facility, but it was too late.

My mother showed up, and I was not allowed to go back with the lady. So I ran away from the facility. A lot of us was going out to the field to do some cheerleader things. I remember and I ran out. I went to Connecticut. I met this man. I lived with him. I told him I was 18 years old. "I am a woman." I made a big lie, so he took me to Connecticut. I was in the newspaper as a missing person. He said, "No, I am not going to jail for you." He dumped me. He threw me out of the house. He was 20 something. I was only 15. From there, I was baby-sitting in Connecticut, and I didn't know how to get back. This lady felt sorry for me, and I said I could baby-sit her two kids. She was going on vacation.

So I saved all my money when she went to Puerto Rico. I went to Puerto Rico with a man and came back with a man. He was 48 years old. I tell you, kids do things. He got killed. He is my oldest son's father. But I had a rough life. He took me to the country there was animals. I didn't know how to deal with that. It was a farm, cows, horses, pigs, squirrels, and chickens. And he hit me.

One time he had one chicken tied at the leg with little chicks and told me, "Dolores, it is time to feed the animals." But I hear the little chick with the mommy. She was in there and I was scared. I knew I was going to be hit. I went over there and she was dead. Oh man, the man beat the living heck out of me. So I said, I deserved it because he told me to watch them. But what could I do? He used to hit me a lot. I had a big mouth though, "I won't stay here." I pick up anything and hit him with it. Then it got to be too much. Too much fighting and the judge went to court.

Even the judge didn't know my age or he would have been jail. They didn't even bother to ask my age, how old I was. He took me to court. I didn't take him to court. I hit him with a hammer in his head. They didn't know he was beating me because I didn't give no complaint. They told me to stay away from him. Not allowed to go to his house. I didn't dare open my mouth and tell them I was homeless. I didn't have no place to live. What was I going to do?

So I had the child and they told him, "You have to give her $7 a week for the child." I got so upset I even cursed the judge. "What the f__am I going to do with $7 and live on the street?"

Dolores was resilient and found a way to survive and care for her infant.

I worked in a bar. It was easy for me to do. They would give me a place to live in the basement. I was allowed to have my children there. I worked in the nighttime, and the daytime I was with my son. I was doing much partying and doing too much drinking. To be in a bar, you have to do what they do in a bar. And then I was sick. I was drinking too much. I was so sick, and I was doing things I was not supposed to do. And then I said, "No." I came back to New York. When my mother saw me, she said, "Oh no!" She was happy, but I wasn't that happy.

Dolores explained how she had held her home as a comfort in her mind all the years she had been away and was so shocked to find it gone. The building had been torn down and her family had moved to a different location; her brother, however, continued to frequent a bar in the old neighborhood. Dolores still desired to be reunited with her family after all she had been through.

When I came over here the building was gone. All those years, the building was going to be there. But there was a bar on the corner that remembered my mother. I asked for my family. And they said they been gone for a long time. He [Dolores's brother] comes around here. He works around here. When my brother saw me, he was so happy. "You're alive." They thought I was dead. It was nice. Then I started on welfare.

When Dolores returned to her family on the East Coast, she was 18, a mother and lost. She was searching for home, stability, and control. Welfare provided food and shelter, but it did not keep her from being pulled into the world of drugs, prostitution, and prison.

REFLECTIONS

Taking a structural perspective, both Betty's and Dolores's stories begin with their mothers in the 1950s and 1960s, when industrial work opportunities and welfare relief led to dominant migration patterns to the Northern states from the Southern states and the islands. Their mothers' transition into a new culture left the families having to respond to more demands from the environment than they could handle. As a result, the childhood and adolescent years of these two participants were harsh, demanding, and appalling. Food and housing insecurity continued to be problems of everyday life for them and their families, and it was not until they became recipients of welfare relief that they could gather some stability to eat on a regular schedule and perhaps live in a particular location for a period of time.

Surviving adversity included developing relationships with maternal or sisterly figures, engaging in legitimate activities and illegitimate activities leading to the path to prison, and ultimately creating an ethic of care for the younger generation. It appears that surviving adversity improved once welfare relief, an external resource, alleviated their hunger. Welfare's structure, such as timely payments and food availability, somewhat reduced family disruption and lack of external controls by bringing families together for meals and creating a basic schedule to ensure family nourishment.

It is this early experience of learning how welfare helped their families that raised their present fears and uncertainty. With the end of welfare and without the skills necessary to sustain employment, the participants were facing many of the same issues in their own families that they had faced in the past, and they wondered how they would continue to survive adversity.

doi:10:1300/J004v23n03_06

Chapter 7

Workfare: Day to Day

SUMMARY. In this chapter, I present the participants' experiences in the work setting from their own perspective. doi:10.1300/J004v23n03_07 [*Article copies available for a fee from The Haworth Document Delivery Service: 1-800-HAWORTH. E-mail address: <docdelivery@haworthpress.com> Website: <http://www.HaworthPress.com> © 2007 by The Haworth Press, Inc. All rights reserved.*]

KEYWORDS. Workfare, nursing home, GED, new learning, employment, reassessment

INTRODUCTION

All participants were in their second or third year of the program, except for Connie, who had just started workfare and was relatively new at the nursing home. By this time, as volunteers in the nursing home, they had learned some important realities. They were aware that the facility was being paid for the volunteers' participation as part of the workfare program agreement with the nursing home. Large numbers of volunteers

---

[Haworth co-indexing entry note]: "Workfare: Day to Day." Greer, Ellen. Co-published simultaneously in *Occupational Therapy in Mental Health* (The Haworth Press, Inc.) Vol. 23, No. 3/4, 2007, pp. 87-126; and: *Women's Immersion in a Workfare Program: Emerging Challenges for Occupational Therapists* (Ellen Greer) The Haworth Press, 2007, pp. 87-126. Single or multiple copies of this article are available for a fee from The Haworth Document Delivery Service [1-800-HAWORTH, 9:00 a.m. - 5:00 p.m. (EST). E-mail address: docdelivery@haworthpress.com].

participated in the program, and they realized they would not be hired by the nursing home, even though they had reported having been promised that, after several months, they would get a job at their workfare placement. It also had become clear that although specialized training programs had been promised, such promises could not be fulfilled, such as the in-house program for nurse's aide certification. When training opportunities were offered, basic resources such as transportation and baby-sitting money were denied, making it impossible to take advantage of the training.

Finally, unpredictable mishaps in the system occurred. For example, throwing a person off the roster left the person without any resources, or, when it came to reassignment, there was no guarantee of being placed in a position that would build on the skills already learned in previous assignments.

Given these problems, the participants described how they adapted to uncertain circumstances. Their stories illustrate how they sometimes found much good in their workfare experiences–learning new skills, finding a supervisor willing to teach, and learning to care for and understand a difficult population. In coping with more negative experiences, the participants struggled to gain respect and recognition, faced the hopelessness of not getting hired and not getting enough education, and combating exhaustion from their daily labor activities with the nursing home residents. These volunteers usually maintained their goal of getting off welfare, finding a good paying job, and becoming more literate–for themselves and their families.

Below are the workfare stories of Florence, Agnes, Connie, Dolores, Esther, and Betty.

FLORENCE: I'M ALMOST THERE

Florence aspired to go as far as she possibly could in the field of nursing. Born into a family of nurses, she was aware of the consistent employment that nursing afforded. She viewed a career in nursing "as a way to go" because it contained all the elements of a job she required as a single mother: stability, livable salary, benefits, and flexible hours.

Her attitude towards her workfare assignments was positive.

> *This program has enabled me to get experience in the field that I want to work in. It has helped me get out there, meet people, stuff like that. Here at the nursing home, I am learning basically what the job is of the certified nursing assistant, which I am going to school for, and basically it has been a great help to me because as*

much as you have your certificate, it is required that you have an
amount of experience in certain facilities for you to get hired.

She valued her workfare experiences as building blocks to her chosen career. She hoped that a resume reflecting her latest assignments, together with recommendations from the site, would lead to gaining a position as a certified nursing assistant. The previous year, she had received her GED, and she then participated in an evening training program to become a certified nurse's assistant. She had completed the coursework, and all she needed was the $115 to pay for the certification exam.

MEETING GOALS WITH THE HELP
OF NURSING SUPERVISORS

Florence's goal in the work setting was to get hands-on experience. One way to accomplish that was to gain the favor of nursing supervisors who were willing to teach her and let her try nursing activities independently.

If I do get the chance to do a little more, the nurses have confi-
dence in me, which I am really happy about. Basically, I come in
and start making beds. That needs to be done. If certain patients
have not yet finished their breakfasts, I will assist them, or if the
nurses need assistance, they just need a second person there while
their cleaning or changing a patient, dressing a patient, washing a
patient, stuff like that. I will do that to assist them, transfer, which
is like moving from bed to chair or chair to bed, stuff like that.

Florence was grateful to the nurses whom she met at the hospital where she had been assigned, just prior to this nursing home assignment. When she had first begun at the hospital, she had been nervous and wondered if she could do the work. She threw herself into her work and discovered that the nursing staff viewed her in a good light. New opportunities emerged from her working relationships with the hospital nurses.

There was a nurse at the hospital, like a supervisor. She put me to
work. She was very nice. She let me help her, and I assisted and she
would come in and say, "very nice work." She would come in and
see how I did. A couple of times, they gave me a patient to take care
of wash up and stuff like that, but no medication, I'm not allowed
to do that. They were very pleased with my work. There I worked

on different floors, wherever I was needed, so I had a wide range of nurses. They would say, "This nurse is asking for you to come on their floor this morning," so I guess I did a good job. It was most everyone, but Marie was really the one who told everyone, "I will send Florence. She is really good." She gave me confidence. I was doing okay. She was very nice, and if I need a reference or anything, she gave me her name and her number. A patient was going home, and she recommended me to the family.

BREAKING IN AT THE NURSING HOME

Initially when Florence was assigned to the nursing home, she had to work hard to find nurses willing to work with her, as well as establish boundaries of respect because of her status as a welfare volunteer.

They (the staff) look down on you. Knowing the kind of person you are is the basis of getting people to look at you for who you are and not what they perceive you to be if you are on public assistance. A lot of the nurses here are very nice. Most of the nasty ones are not on this floor anyway. I don't have to really interact with them anyway, but a couple of times they come down here and you hear how they talk.

I am not a volunteer that come in and no, I guess judge you like the rest or until they get to know you different. It takes about two weeks until they get to know you. I guess it all depends on where they come from. They see that you come here and don't want to do nothing, and they treat you like a person that don't want to do anything. If you treat them with respect, I guess they treat you with respect. You also have to let them know that you are not going to take any bullshit, too. I like to say to myself, if a person doesn't like me as a person, they cannot say I come here and I don't do my part. So they have to give me respect. If nothing else, they have to give me that. They cannot go and tell the supervisor that this girl, she don't do anything 'cause people will find every little thing on you when they don't like you, but if they don't like you, that is their personal thing.

I had a person attack me, and I surprised myself 'cause I took it quite calmly, and I guess when they saw, they expected me to feel bad and attack back I didn't. After that it was okay. But it all depends. If I do something wrong, I would say it. I'm the kind of person that is not going to take my problems out on anyone.

MAKING MISTAKES CAN PROVIDE NEW LEARNING

Florence was not only open with how she related to others if she was wrong, but she was finding out that working with patients was not easy and that she made mistakes. Finding a way to frame this type of learning by contrasting changes in herself helps integrate her experience of learning about the needs of others.

> *I am learning about understanding. I am not going to do every-thing the way I am supposed to cause I can slip up and do some-thing or assume that somebody wants when they really don't. Even yesterday, there is a lotion they put on the patient. I didn't know she doesn't like that lotion on her skin. Now I know she doesn't like that lotion. So I was getting to understand the patients, their likes and dislikes without taking it personally. Like Dorothea was say-ing, these are patients and they have their problems. They are go-ing to be nasty at times, and you have to understand it is part of the training. That we have to understand how they are. Even me. I used to be a lot thinner. I could run down the block, and now I can't even run too hard. I'm puffing and huffing. Things you used to do you can't do. Our bodies change as we get older, you know. It is part of the understanding.*

IT'S A HEAVY LOAD

Eventually Florence began to talk about how tiring the work was.

> *The job is a heavy load. Taking care of a lot of patients. It's basi-cally stressful. I'm tired when I get home, and I don't have the pa-tience to do things with my children. I might want to do in the evening try to help them with their homework. I really try my best, but by the end of the day I'm beat. I think the stressful part is getting the rest you need. If you don't get that rest, you're not physically or mentally ready to do your job. Lack of sleep will make anybody ag-gravated and agitated and miserable. That I feel is the worst part about not getting enough rest.*

Although she was tired, she was a model volunteer and earned respect from several members of the nursing staff. When she disappeared from the nursing home in the early winter, there was a rumor that Florence had found a job. Everyone found this believable, in addition to wanting it to be true because of her high level of performance.

BEING CUT OFF

What really happened, however, shocked everyone. When her cycle at the nursing home was completed, Florence had not received a letter to inform her of her new assignment. Instead, her benefits were unexpectedly cut off. She had to leave the nursing home. After some time, she was reassigned to do sanitation activities in a housing development, but she refused this assignment because it did not meet her needs in developing a nursing career profile. During the period of appeal, she had no benefits, and waiting for a new assignment and reinstitution of her benefits created a financial crisis. Although she lived with her aunt, she was responsible for her half of the rent and for providing resources for her three children. She feared breaking down emotionally, but she coped by refraining her circumstances.

Some people don't deserve certain things to happen to them. But then again, bad things happen to you and you don't know why. But it could be for the good, for the better. Like all this waiting I am going through now. I am praying it is for the better. I am trying not to look at it as a downfall. I am just praying that all this waiting is not in vain, you know. And If I don't make it, I will probably bug out, and I don't have time for that. I have three children, and they don't need a crazy mother, you know.

During the months of waiting for a reassignment, she made the best of a bad situation.

To tell you the truth, I could be home again, you know, because these months I have been working have been hard. I am glad in a sense that I am home with my children. A few things happened at the end of the school year, like my daughter had a stepping up ceremony and I was able to go. Stuff I done with them that I couldn't have done if I was at work.

When financial problems become a burden, Florence was confident that her spiritual relationship with God would be a source of assistance.

If I didn't have financial problems, everything would be okay, but mostly that is what makes people bug out, you know. My mother was this much away from a nervous breakdown, and I am not going to let that happen to me. I used to trip a lot: "God, I have to pay this bill. Where will I get the money from?" They have this thing they send you from welfare. If I live in the same place for some time, they send you back $65 as an incentive. That check has come to me at times. Like I have tomorrow to pay a bill, and they might cut it off, and I will go to the mailbox today and find that check And I say, "Thank you Lord." So he finds a way for me. Like my friend came up with a job for me for just two weeks, but it really kept my head above water.

NO JOB IS TOO FAR WHEN YOU'RE DESPERATE

Florence was able to earn money for two weeks during the time she was off the welfare roster. Her friend had referred her for a private homecare case to help a man who was quite ill. To reach his home every day, Florence had to travel many hours.

Let me tell you how desperate I was when my friend got me that job. It was in Rivington. I had to take three trains and a bus to get there. It took me two hours to get there and two hours to get back. I had to leave my house at 6am to get there at 8am. I always said Rivington is too far for me. Manhattan is far enough for me, but I was desperate for that money, and I got up every morning and went to Rivington. I would leave there at 4pm and go straight to the school and pick up my kids at 6pm after school.

Implied in Florence's situation are the changes she needed to make in child-care, especially the morning routines. Fortunately, she lived with a relative who helped her get the children dressed, fed, and off to school during that time.

Working with her new patient was challenging for Florence. She provided necessary but labor-intensive care, including changing his colostomy bag, packing an infected wound with sterile gauze and saline solution, changing his sheets, rolling him over and back, and keeping him company. She evaluated the experience:

I will say that going out on these jobs has benefited me on how I move. I get things done faster. I am more organized. When you are home, you don't think about this stuff I learn from these people.

PREPARING FOR FUTURE EMPLOYMENT: DON'T BURN BRIDGES

In reflecting on her experiences, Florence was proud that she had left every position on good terms and with a recommendation. While she waited for a new assignment, she commented about considering asking Camilla, the supervisor at the nursing home, for a reference.

In life when you are young, you don't know that a lot of what you do can come back to haunt you. Thank God I haven't burned too many bridges behind me. This is my aim right now. I go to the job fair and some of them look at you like they expect us to fail, but I don't care. I am there to do a job, and I am going to do it. Whether I am getting paid for it or not, that is me. I am going to do the job so tomorrow if I have to ask that nurse to recommend me for something. That is my way. The more I do, the more I learn. I do a few things I'm not supposed to do, but I'm not going to go overboard and get myself in trouble. I want to help. I am helping them and they are helping me. The nurses were glad for our help. They encourage you, and you need to hear that sometimes too. You don't want to go there and hear you're butterfingers and they shouting at you and getting in trouble.

Florence valued reciprocity and recognition in her working relationships. Being cooperative with others and also accepting her own need for positive validation seemed to help guide her in her overall career plan. She did, however, see problems with the program in relation to choice, consistency of assignments, and the need to develop sensitivity toward immigrant women who may be working for the first time.

My problem is with the whole welfare system. They need to have more programs for people in fields that they want to work in. I don't see that you take people and shove them into any job and then send them to five different jobs. The only time I could choose was when I finished PEP and went to START. Then I went to FIRST START and

I went to school. I was in school for nursing, and I saw that they had hospitals, and I chose to go to those hospitals. That's why I'm willing to do the work that I am doing, because I chose to do it.

I believe they should have more programs like that where they can choose this nurse's aide program. All the money they wasting, they can have a nurse's aide school and send them out to jobs. Instead, they send them out to different jobs, one day clerical and the next cleaning the streets. How are you supposed to get a job when these are things you're supposed to put on a resume? These things, clerical, to cleaning the streets to doing something in a hospital or doing childcare. A lot of the girls are working in day care centers. And they themselves tell you an employer looks at that, and they see that you are an unstable person. They see your jobs are from one field to the next. How do you tell your employer it is not your fault, welfare sent you from one place to another?

Carrying the stigma of welfare was a concern for Florence, and many of her peers agreed that when they went on interviews, they did not want to reveal that the work experience reflected on their résumés was workfare related. Other concerns about getting hired were fears of discrimination of age, race, and immigrant status.

I had to do something before I reach a certain age where nobody wants to hire me. You know it is rough. Maybe race plays apart in it too, but I think it has to do more with stereotypical truths that they have about people on welfare, that they are lazy, they don't want to do this. I mean, one bad apple spoils the whole bunch. I think that if they try to move away from the stereotypes and try to talk to people that are ignorant out there, yes, there are ones who come and don't want to do nothing, but that is not everybody. Most people come, they can't speak English and that is a problem for them. They are at an age where they are scared to try something new.

It is hard if you are from another country. Just trying to get used to another way of life, and then there are women who have never worked a day in their lives and it is scary for them. They think they are not smart enough, they don't have the intelligence, they don't think they can do it. And they need that push. They have a few classes, which sort of like therapy, talk to teach you

*how to be, how to do this, how to get a job. We know there is a
language barrier.*

Florence had empathy for the barriers her immigrant peers faced. Her
own immigration from England made her know how difficult the transition to a new culture could be. She seemed to advocate for a workfare program that addressed the individual needs and opportunities for free choice
of work assignments.

At the time of the last interview when I met with Florence in her home,
she was waiting for a new assignment and had to put off sitting for her certification exam until she could save up the required fee.

AGNES: I'M 100% SERIOUS

Between caring for her father when he was seriously ill and her daily
experience at the nursing home working with patients, Agnes felt prepared to be a home health aide. Her only obstacle was that she needed a
certificate, but her workfare schedule did not allow her the time to take
the course that was required for the certificate. Without the START program's approval to attend the training course instead of appearing at her
workfare assignment, Agnes would jeopardize her welfare benefit.
There was not enough time to take a course even between workfare cycles. There was such a great need for nurse's aide training, and many of
the volunteers were making a request to have a special program designed for them.

*Since they see a lot of people want to go into the home health, they
thinking about getting a program together so we can get the certificate and a job that way. The START lady said that she was going
to bring in a worker last week but it hasn't happened yet. When I
see it, I'll believe it.*

BROKEN PROMISES

Agnes had good reason to be skeptical.

*They said when the program first started, it was six months and
then you were guaranteed a job. Then people who did six months
came back and did another six months. People have been here two
or three years and they haven't got a job yet.*

*When summertime comes, they pay summer youth to do the same
thing. They could just hire us. I'm not saying summer youth don't
need work that teach them how to go about business-wise. Since
they find job openings for them, they could find them for us 'cause
summer youth are only doing it for the summertime and we need it
full time. We have families to feed. They bring summer youth in
during the summertime and pay them, and we still get just carfare
and baby-sitting money.*

Agnes was angry. She felt a sense of injustice over the volunteers' need
to get jobs not being recognized and their not being treated the same as the
young people in the summer program. She saw the importance of giving
the young people opportunities but could not understand why the volunteers were not hired to earn a salary. Getting off welfare was a priority. She
had already passed her GED and was considering home health or nursing
as a potential area for work. Agnes's interest in becoming a professional
caregiver stemmed from her working with Alice, a patient with Parkinson's
disease.

AGNES AND ALICE

Alice's condition was deteriorating. She needed to be in a padded room
to prevent fractures from her repeated falls. Always agitated, even in the
reclining geri-chair, Alice often became calmer under Agnes's care. Every morning Agnes arrived at Alice's room ready to braid her hair. One
day I joined them and noticed that Alice looked content as Agnes braided
Alice's hair.

*As long as I am around her, she is content. She got so attached to
me. That's my second mother, right Alice? (Alice replies, "yeah.")
She has kids. They come and see her, but she is ready to go
home. Kids work and no one is home, and she has to be watched
constantly or she will fall and hurt herself. But she don't want to
hear that. She just wants to go home. I guess that's where I come in
because I stay until five o'clock and stay with her. So she sees me
as her daughter. So even when her daughter came here to feed her,
I told her I been telling Alice that she was coming the next day, but
Alice started crying 'cause she don't have nobody but me sitting
right there feeding her.*

They say when the daughter is here and she wants to do something, the daughter says, "Oh mama, please," and walks away or something like that. I be doing more attention than the daughter is doing.

Agnes was very sensitive to Alice's need for care and attention and understood the significance a daughter's role can play in a mother's care. Her own mother was recently recovering from a stroke, and Agnes helped with her mother's care. Agnes acknowledges the relationship between her empathy for her mother, for Alice, and for all the residents who yearn for their families to take them home:

I braid her hair, talk to her, sit with her, feed her. Some other people in here when you ask them to do their hair, just box braid it, but it still doesn't look combed, so it doesn't make sense. I know if it was my mother, I would want her appearance to look neat. So that is why I take my time with them because I know how I want my mother to look and how her hair to look. I do theirs the same way I do my daughter's or my mother. When they are done and thinking about their family, and when they want to go home, it takes a while for them to get cheered back up. I try to make them laugh, kiss them, give them a hug every now and then.

CONSIDERING OTHER OCCUPATIONS

Agnes was dedicated to giving the best care. For a while, she looked forward to the promise of a home health aid course at the nursing home, but it never materialized. She heard about a new program called "Women's Talents" that trained women in nontraditional occupations.

You can learn construction and electrician work at Women's Talents. They make like 11 and up, 11 to 17 per hour. One lady said doing the engineer work cleaning the train made 12 per hour. Just picking up the trash off the train tracks. They got maintenance where you can plaster and fix things. I believe they had the home health training, too.

Agnes hoped she could transition to Women's Talents when her cycle at the nursing home was completed, but she had yet to experience any support from the Start Program in providing the necessary training.

Most of the programs tell you there are night programs out there. That what you do with your spare time if you want to get on. A lot of them is nasty, like the money is coming out of their pockets. They don't care you're on or off. They just don't want to deal with you at times. I guess you'll be homeless if you haven't found anything by then 'cause they want to eliminate it all together, 'cause they aren't really worried if your kids eat 'cause they eating.

Agnes expresses how she must care for herself in order to make it. Like Florence, she contrasts herself to others who do not try hard.

You have to care for yourself. You have to work your tail off to learn the skills in the different places you go. That's why you have to make sure some of them play games. They go to the doctor, get the note they were sick, but were sitting home and watching stories, whatever. Some of them, and they are not serious. Whatever programs they send me to, I am 100% serious about the program. Whatever skills you are giving me, I am going to take in. When I leave, I will have those skills with me.

RESPECT IN RELATIONSHIPS WITH OTHERS

Agnes' assertion that she was 100% serious about the program included her relationships with staff. Respect was an essential ingredient to her interaction with others. She thought every person deserved respect and she expected to be treated with respect, as well.

You know off the bat how I am talking to you is how I expect to be talked to. I respect you. You gonna respect me. I don't care if it is a worker or someone sitting at a desk giving me a paper, a man, a president himself giving me money in his hand. That is how you will talk to me and see me. Some of them talk down to you any kind of way.

The "them" to whom Agnes was referring were the supervisors and staff with whom she had worked in the workfare program. At the nursing home, she found a sense of fairness:

Here at the nursing home, the ones downstairs [Dorothea] tell you, "I am the same as you. I was on Welfare and found a way to

get off." They let you know so don't try to take advantage of me
and tell me or I couldn't make it 'cause of this, 'cause sometimes
they let you get over. Everyday you got to do what you got to do
'cause if you come every day and do what you got to do, you can go
to them and say, "I need to leave today," and they say, "Make sure
you bring documentation." You bring back that documentation,
and they let you sign in for the day. But if you play games, they
know you playing game. You not ready for anything. All you want
to do is sit back and collect the money.

Many of the volunteers are supportive of one another if they are
not into themselves. Some of them is just into getting all the jewelry
and clothing their men have bought them. They think they better
than you because they dress better than you. Most of the jobs I had
were okay because we worked together.

Agnes got along with the other volunteers. Most often she would be
found sitting with Alice. After several months, Agnes began to mention
that the stress of caring for her mother and the ill patients at the nursing
home was becoming too much. She did not want to become a home health
aide after all. It was too depressing watching the residents cry during holiday time. Clearly, Agnes was sensitive to loss and sadness.

You get close to them and then they pass. Then someone else you
have to get close to and then hope they don't pass. But this is their
last stop in the nursing home, you know, and it bound to happen
sooner or later. Now I am trying to focus on my mother. Taking
care of her. That the only thing that be on my mind right now.

As mentioned earlier, Agnes had decided to take the Women's Talent
Program, hoping that the training would lead to a job with a major utility
company that paid a livable wage. She had some ideas of how the
workfare program could be improved. When she added up her benefit, she
noticed that it was the same amount as a regular job, so she suggested that
workfare become a regular job with a regular weekly paycheck. She commented on how waiting every three weeks for a check in the present
system with the occasional system breakdowns made it very hard to manage her finances.

You want everybody to get off welfare; it cost a lot of money. Pay
every week so you can budget it down like a paying job. You are
paying the people [businesses] because the people that is taking

the volunteers, they [Welfare] is giving them a stipend to put them in their place of business or wherever they are at, so that money could be going to a pay check. Like I said, it is going to end in five years. There is not going to be any volunteers doing it for free. So make these real jobs.

In January, Agnes left the nursing home to join the Women's Talents' Program.

CONNIE: A WOMAN NEEDS TO HAVE BACKBONE

Connie was a single mother of three children. Whenever she talked with me, she mentioned how she looked forward to the day that she could tell her children she had a job. It was not easy facing the uncertainty that a job might not be there after her workfare experience. She began to believe that the only way to move ahead and become a professional woman was to enter a college program.

I take the training and try to make the best that I can to my ability, to see I get hired, which I doubt, since I've been in this program six months. I have tried my best and seen that I don't miss one day. I don't see anything working out for me. I've decided to go to school. I am hoping that while I'm in school I will learn a trade to get a job and stand on my feet. Since I've been in the program, I haven't seen anything. It is like going in a circle.

In the Start Program, you go to work Monday, Tuesday, Wednesday, then you're on job search Friday, going to the stores looking for a job or any interviews. You don't get hired. Some places say if you don't have an education, they can't hire you. I haven't seen anything so far. That is why I decided I want to go to school for nurse's aide. I have been here and I already have the training. I just need the studies. I am going to put a lot of effort because I want to do something for myself. You know, I want my kids to be proud of me. That is what I am really looking forward to. First of all, I want to get my GED. That is what I am really aiming for. I was in a GED program. I did very well. There was a teacher who was willing to help me with math tutoring. He sent me work over the mail. I send him work over the mail, and he checks it. I gave him a call and he gave me the worksite where the GED is being taken. I think I'm ready. Let's see what happens. After the GED, I want to take up mental health or nutritionist to see if I make it. That will be like a step up. Then I will work my way through. My goal is to have a job to support myself and support my family, have a profession, so with my kids I can sit down with them and say, no matter how old I was, I got this and I want you to try to do better than I did.

Connie enjoyed her work with the elderly at the nursing home. Learning how to work with the older residents inspired her to want to continue her education in mental health.

I learned how to communicate with the elderly. It is not easy. I learned what is their needs, what they want. I learned how to be in an environment with them. They need care. They feel lonely. I am going to get to that age soon, and I want someone to treat me good. The training I got here is how to be in an environment, how to understand them and see if I can help them. I would like to. That is why I want to take mental health.

How did Connie learn so much about communicating with the elderly? Her assignment was to visit a nursing home resident in his/her room twice a day to talk with or read to the resident. Camilla called this activity "motivation," and she had some of the volunteers assigned to specific residents. Through this daily activity, Connie learned other tasks related to their care. She developed a philosophy of how she wanted to be helpful in the work environment and could translate the therapeutic impact of her work on others and then apply it to her own life.

I learned also how to make beds and feed. I love feeding them. I like motivating them. I really like motivation. If you don't get motivated, you stay down. A lot of the girls say so much personal problems. But you come in here smiling. And I say, if I let my personal problems rise, then I am down. What good is that for me because I have children? You know what I do? I apply it to myself. I say when I am down, you got to go to work. You come through that door. You leave your private life outside that door. You come in here and do a job.
One thing I learned, you either come in here and work. You try to be as courteous as you can. You mind your business. You don't get into other people's business. I feel that if you come here and I say good morning, and if I can help you with anything, I would. But as getting along, I am not a hard person to get along with. I like to give love to see if I can get it back. If you don't want to be

bothered. I won't bother you. But I will try to say good morning, good afternoon. Some people I just say hi to, they just look at me.

The nurse upstairs, the one in the dayroom, I love working with her. She is such a wonderful person. She is likable. She gives you strength to want to work with them. The rest of them I don't bother. I see if you don't want to be bothered, I don't bother you. I don't have any problems. I haven't had, thank God.

Connie often thought about how her life would have been different if she had finished high school.

I have cried many days coming to work here. If only I had listened to my mother [crying], going to school and doing what I was supposed to do, I wouldn't be like this right now. I know I am not going to let this get me down [workfare]. I am going to get back up on my feet, and I am thinking, should I go to school or stay in the program? So I pray, "God, what should I do? You tell me what to do." He always tells me what to do. I always say, God has me here for a purpose because what I didn't get, he wants me to give to someone else. I am going to do that, to be a professional. Mental health? I'm not healed from that experience of losing my baby, and you need to be. I think we women have to be strong. I don't know. These are my grandmother's words. You have to be strong backbone. You have to think what you are going to see yourself somewhere.

Connie shared her vision of how she saw herself working in the future.

I see myself in a hospital or in a nursing home. I see myself very busy, and I see myself working with patients, and that is what gets me motivated.

While working in the nursing home, Connie was cooperative and sought opportunities to keep busy.

I am a person who likes to keep busy. I come into the day room in the morning. I do motivational rounds. If that person is not in their room or the dayroom, I know that they are in the hospital. I worry how is Ms. Glenworth. Ms. Glenworth is very sick. Wow, let me see if I could send her a card. When I finish bringing the residents into the dayroom, I run into the physical therapy room. "Do you need me to transport anyone upstairs?" and they say, "Thank-you."

That's me. I keep myself busy. I make friends with the staff some of the nurses are very nice, and some of them treat you bad because you're a volunteer. I tell them, "I am not a volunteer. I am an intern." That is how they treat us. Less! I don't let that get to me; a lot of the girls here have that on their mind. We have to be called "volunteer." We love to be called "intern." It is a professional word. These people don't use that. Call me "volunteer" and I won't answer you. My paper says " internship." See, you have to learn to be professional. I don't have all my education, but I try to apply what I learned in school. You know, I figure, if you got a job you got to be a professional at it, and that is what I am doing. I am going back to college. This is my best bet. Look at those girls upstairs. They don't know what they want to do. When your time is up, you go to the TAR Program and means that you can go to sanitation or you could work sweeping the streets. That is why I have been thinking and I said to myself, I am not falling into that situation. I'm not. I'm not.

REASSESSMENT

Connie's hopes to start school that winter never were fulfilled. At the end of January, her cycle was up at the nursing home, and she was prepared to start a new assignment. Instead, she received a letter mandating her to start all over in reassessment. This translated into having to start the entire process from the beginning. Making the situation more problematic, the letter had been initially sent to the wrong address, so for a period of time, Connie had no idea of her status. Once she was notified, there was no room for her in the next reassessment group. She stayed home for three weeks and, during that time, searched for a job and realized how difficult it is to obtain employment. Connie described how she coped:

I stood home three weeks doing nothing, depressed, couldn't find a job. Outside everything is hard. What did I do? I kept myself busy. I did a lot of reading and stuff a lot of job sites, going over, seeing if they needed me, and I volunteer, you know. Finally, I was rescheduled to start the 22nd of February. I started there, and on the first day I didn't like it.

Connie returned to the main office, where a large orientation program for new workfare participants was held. At the beginning, she disliked the group leader, but as she allowed herself to become involved in the process of the activities, she not only learned new information, but she changed her attitude toward the leader. The orientation period also gave her an opportunity to mentor new group members.

> *By the end of the week, that person [group leader] I give a lot of thanks to. First, she gave out cards. Whatever you pick. tragedy— you talk about your image. If you pick hearts—is love, you talk about your passion. If you pick club—tragedy. If you pick diamond—I think it is your efforts. I don't really remember all of them. I know I got tragedy. The first thing I did was get up there. I was so nervous. When I got up there, I said my name was Connie. I said I am in the Start Program and I am happy to be back because I was depressed being home and not doing nothing. When I was in Start, I was motivated. I was working. I was going to school. You know, I felt my life back on track. My tragedy was my grandmother passed, and I asked Start if I could travel with my mother to the funeral, and they said, no because I was to be rescheduled. It hurt, but I just let the wind take it away. So what happened after that, I just sat down and then what happened. I learned about résumes, and I learned about how to present yourself when you go on an interview.*
>
> *I learned so many things in that first orientation, and I didn't like the leader because she was rude and nasty, but I understood what point she was coming from. That's why I gave her my undivided attention because I wanted . . . . You see, there are things about her that I want to apply to my life. Sometimes you have to speak to an adult in a harsh way so they wake up and know that this is reality. You know, I am happy that I pass and then I came back here to my job site. The first day I came in I had regrets 'cause there was a little misunderstanding, and I learned to cope with it. I want to be here [at the nursing home] or am I here 'cause there are no job sites available. I start thinking and I said any job you get you going to have to learn to deal with people's attitudes, behavior. There are so many different kinds of people at all levels. You have to learn and that is what I did.*

FEAR OF REJECTION

Part of the learning for Connie was coming to grips with identifying the fear associated with getting a job.

The biggest fear is getting rejected from a job because of color, race, or language. I said to myself, well, I am sorry I got an accent. I know that I am from another country and know that I don't have an education. This is one thing I ain't going to let that beat me. I got up and said, "I am sorry. I go into my job site every morning. I could be depressed from stress, from my children, from owing bills, but I am going to come into the nursing home. I am going to show my face, even if I have to fake it. I am going to show I am coming to work. Even if I don't get paid, I am going to come because I have that experience. I could take that to the next level." That is what I learned, you have to pick up and continue. And this is what I am doing.

HOW TO MAKE IT: DON'T BE AFRAID

She shared her perspective on how to cope with fear with the new workfare participants at the orientation. She felt she understood the fears they expressed in the workshop and wanted to help them prepare for their first assignment.

Since I was already in the program and I already knew about it, I said, "Listen, go into the job site and show them that you are willing, ask them how you can help them. You help them in anything they need you for and make sure you don't miss a lot of days. If you have important things, always let them know."

When we would get a break, we used to sit down and talk. That was their first time and this was my third time around. I told them there is nothing to be afraid of, to think positive. I explained how to fill out time sheets, how to report, how to fax them, and then they feel calm. There was another girl, she felt sad because she came out of a drug rehab and she said she was afraid to go back into society. She was afraid she would be rejected because she did bad things and had her children taken away. I told her, "Listen, everybody had a bad day." I cannot sit here and say, "You took drugs." No, I have a worse skeleton in my closet than she might have. I don't judge people. Like I said, I don't judge people no more. What's in your heart, that's how you are. That's what I learn. I motivated people because for me too it is like a therapy for me. Well, I say, "Don't be afraid. If you got that problem, face it." I learned this because my grandmother taught me this.

WE ARE ALL IN THE SAME SHOE

When Connie returned to the nursing home, she experienced more conflict with Camilla; however, she also became more aware of her own attitudes and the necessity for the volunteers to work together, not only to get the tasks completed, but also as a protection from punitive authority. She talked about the internal conflict between the volunteers:

> *We all come here with attitudes. We all come here and we don't want to do things. Well, I am not talking about myself, but I am talking about what I learned from the girls. We all get along because we all understand we are in the same shoe. Teamwork is the thing I learned. When we come here in the morning, there is nobody over nobody. All work as a team. We pair up in groups now. We works as a team, and if we cannot get along, we lock ourselves up in a room and say, "Watch your behavior" and watch our tone to find a way to work around. That is and so. Let me call her up. Everybody has everybody's number. When you don't come to work, I am calling you to find out if you're okay. Is there something I can help you with on the floor? We are like a family.*
>
> *There are people here with different attitudes like, "You're not my boss." Those are the attitudes you get when you come in here, and "She didn't tell me to do this." When I first came here, I asked the girls what do I have to do because they were here before me. They told me, "Not really anything. All I need you to do is help me." We need to bring the patients into the dayroom, and then we sit down at lunchtime and ask how many children do you have. We talk about children, how is everything at home, and then we started talking and we bonded. We became a family. When we have a problem, we act like a team. We sit down and talk like a group, like me and Esther.* [Connie recreating the conversation]

Esther.   *I don't like what you are doing. You are sleeping.*
Connie: *I am tired because I didn't get sleep last night.*
Esther: *I can understand that.*
Connie: *Let me go into the back wet my face and freshen up and come back and give you a hand.*

This is how we are. We do not go to the supervisor. She don't want to help me If she says, "She is sleeping." It is unprofessional. Cover your backs and that is what we call team work here.

When I mentioned the metaphor "flowers yearning to bloom" that I thought about in relation to the potential of the volunteers, Connie agreed. She said that she was saying the same thing, just in different words: *"We are willing and wanting, but not getting a chance."* I asked her what would help the volunteers to bloom. She replied, *"Time to grow."*

Esther: *What are they going to do to us?*

Esther did not like the work at the nursing home. Initially, she had wanted to work in housekeeping, and she had been assigned to work in the basement to fold the residents' laundered clothing. Interactions with other workers upset her, as did the lack of ventilation, so she asked Camilla to be reassigned. She was moved to the second-floor dayroom, where Dolores was the head workfare volunteer. The mix of volunteers working in the dayroom suited Esther, but she did not like working with the sick residents and, overall, she felt the time she spent at the nursing home was an obstacle to gaining an education.

> *Really, in this program, there is nothing important because we really are not getting nothing out of it. Like they got us coming in here for six months telling us they are going to give us a job. People have been here for two years and haven't been given a job. So, I don't know what you are going to get out of this program. For me, it is like the schooling is good for me because I am really behind in my school.*
> *I don't like the idea of them working here telling us we are getting a job, 'cause, come on, there are people here for six months. You do six months, then you're back at the same place, and they're starting all over again. What is that? I have to go out there and look myself. We sitting here coming to a place working for free, doing jobs the nurses are supposed to do. I don't think that's fair.*
> *I wanted housekeeping when I first came here. There was a lot of gossip, talking a lot of junk down there. I didn't like it. They moved me up here. Talking to the supervisor of this place, we ain't going to get no job here, so it don't make no sense for us being here. It's just that we are working for nothing. I'm going to stick it out for the time being until I find something.*

THEY DON'T GIVE US NO KIND OF CREDIT

Although Esther did not like the work, she was reliable and helped her fellow volunteers carry out their activities for the residents in the dayroom. She felt demoralized because Camilla, the supervisor, did not appreciate the volunteers' efforts.

Camilla treats us–if you do something right, it ain't enough. She come up here and blow your head off for something she told you to do. When the nurses heard what she was saying down there, how the nurses got their own ideas, she says, "Fix up your room, the day room, until you are able to bring patients inside." She walk up here and we sitting here and got the room all fixed up and she blowup. Something she just told us to do. You come downstairs and say, "Camilla, listen, the patients are not changed or nothing, so we can't do nothing," or "the nurses are not there or something."

They gave us a list of do's and don'ts when we first came here: You cannot sit in that dayroom without a nurse in there. But you're standing out there because it is not ready, yet she comes up and she gets upset with you. "Why are you getting upset with me when you tell me I can not bring these patients in the day room." They make us feel that we do nothing. She can walk up and we're standing in the wrong position because they are not ready for us to do what we are supposed to do. She calls a big meeting. Tells the second floor they are not doing what they supposed to be doing. You know, it makes you feel like, what are they bossing my behind for?

When we first came, we used to bathe the patients. I mean, we used to do a lot. I used to sit in here and feed the patients before I went to lunch. I used to help the nurses hold them up while they were being changed. It's like we don't do nothing. I do what I'm supposed to do. They don't give us no kind of credit.

I don't help the nurses like I used to because we staying and they tell us we doing nothing. They ain't going to make me feel like that. Why do anything? Camilla is like she paying you out of her own pocket. She looks down on us.

The things she says out of her mouth I could tell you she look down on people. One of the girls upstairs, Mona–Dorothea went to Mona's mother's shop, and Dorothea came back and told Camilla how nice it was, and how much stuff the mother had. Camilla said, "Why Mona is so poor. She's on welfare." Why would you say that? Because that is her mother's shop. But Dorothea was telling

*her that her father is still alive, so that is probably his stuff. Why
she got to be poor? Why you ask why she is poor and on welfare,
because her mother has a shop? That's her mother's shop. That is
her own woman! She asked one of the girls, "How do you buy
Tommy Hilfigger when you on welfare? You know, the little things
she saying hurts your feelings. You know she do it when people is
around. It's messed up.*

Esther was uncomfortable with Camilla's attitude toward the volunteers. Like many of the volunteers, she was unable to verbally express her feelings of demoralization or to ask to be treated with more dignity. The one way volunteers showed Camilla that they were dissatisfied was to give minimal attention to the residents. Camilla depended on the volunteers to carry out activities, so when they passively resisted, she received the message, but it never resolved the hurt feelings of the volunteers.

One day Camilla brought lunch for the volunteers, something she had never done before. At first, the volunteers were appreciative, but then they began discussing why she had done this. Esther noted that when Camilla had taken away their smoking break, they had reacted by not feeding the residents lunch; she believed that Camilla was trying to win them over with the lunch and promising the return of the break so that they would continue to feed the residents at lunch time.

Camilla's relationship with the volunteers disturbed Esther. She had worked hard to complete a drug rehab program and had gotten herself off of crack. She had graduated with a new sense of self-esteem. Yet, her situation in workfare was uncertain and she did not want to undo her accomplishments.

*I like the way I live now. It's hard but I like myself more now than I
did before. You think, how is it going to be when they cut the welfare? What are they really going to do?*

Esther had counted on welfare for survival and could not believe that people would be kicked out if they did not have a job.

*If you really don't have a job, what are we going to do? Some people say they can't just cut welfare out. But you don't know what
they are going to do to us. They are going to do it. But they will
have to help people get a job. They cannot just dump people out in
the street and tell them find a job. It is not easy going out there to
find a job. You may be able to flip burgers, but is that going to take*

care of your rent and your food, stuff like that and your kids? No, it's not. Education is important. That's what I think. If you want to get somewhere, you got to get some training, you know.

Esther worked seasonally at a neighborhood amusement park collecting tickets. She had found it on her own. Without an education, Esther thought that working in an office was not feasible. For her, continuing in the program and going to school two days a week seemed the most logical thing to do. Staying in the program beyond her six-month cycle, that spring Esther experienced serious problems with the welfare system and had not received food stamps for herself or her children for four months. She was exceedingly angry that she was keeping her part of the agreement to work for her benefit, but welfare was not keeping its part to provide the monthly resources that she counted on to provide for her family.

> *You call your worker and you try to get your budget thing straightened out. These people don't want to understand things to take care of, and if you are on welfare, you working for your check and they not giving you the things they supposed to. You doing what they ask of you. How can they get upset when you have to go and take care of things? And then in school, the teacher don't want to hear that. He think that staying in school is more important, but you have to take care of business at home. You have to have food in your house for you and your kids. I feel that if I am working for my check, I have to do that. Nobody is giving me a job right now. You need a high school diploma. That is why I really have stress.*

Many things exacerbated Esther's stress. When she began her workfare assignment, she was reunited with her children and was re-entering her mother role. She was focusing on being there for her children, helping them with their schoolwork and fighting for their medical benefits. Losing the food stamp benefit impeded the everyday stability and management she had accomplished with her children. Paradoxically, when Esther had difficulty getting to work because of diminishing transportation money, the absence would be held against her. The system had no problem sanctioning the volunteers, but it seemed as if no policies existed to punish the system for placing the lives of the volunteers in jeopardy.

When I last spoke with Esther, the welfare system was resolving the food stamp problem after many months.

DOLORES: IT'S LIKE WE'RE DRAFTED

When I met Dolores, she had been in the workfare program for three years and the nursing home was her first assignment. At the beginning, she had found it difficult to adjust to the program:

> *First of all, you have to get up in the morning and look for a new job, learn how to do new jobs, even though you're not getting paid for it.*

She realized that staying home was not going to help her in the future, and, over time, she learned to appreciate the opportunity to attend school and wished that the program placed more of an emphasis on education:

> *In the last six months, they gave me a chance to go back to school. At least I would have liked them to give me more time in school than doing work. But when they close a case and there is no more welfare, there will be no more school because you have to support your family. Take whatever you can about school and go on the weekend.*

BEING THERE FOR YOUR CHILD IS NOT ENOUGH

Dolores had two grown children. Her youngest son was eight years old. She had been happy to be home with him until he began to come home from school with homework and asked his mother for assistance.

> *I was there. I was feeling good I was there for my son. For him, I washed his clothes. I wasn't thinking the right way. Being there is not enough for a child. My child, when he started to go to school, start asking me, "Mommy, help me with my homework." Too bad I don't know how to read or write. Even though he was proud he had a mother, there are other kids' mothers are working and don't have time for the kids. Now I see my son is more proud of me now. He see mommy go to school and mommy go help me do homework and mommy go out to work. He doesn't know if I get paid or not, but I don't want to explain to him that I am working for the check. I want him to grow up. I don't want to mess up his mind. I still have time to come home and do homework with him. At the beginning, it was real hard for me. I come tired. I had to work and go to school. I was so upset they taking the time I had for my kids. But at the end, I am getting better for that. At one*

time, I said the heck with workfare. Then I sat down and realized, how am I going to do that, to sit with him to do homework? Where am I going to sit with him, wind up in a shelter, if they have a shelter, because if I am not on welfare, I cannot pay rent. I cannot buy food. He needs food and he needs shelter. A lot of people on workfare don't think that way until they realize that is the way they have to think.

Some people think all these years we had this free. It is hard for what the workfare gives us to a lot of people is not enough. Add everything up, food stamps, Medicare and the tax money they give you, you can survive then.

I KNOW I WILL MAKE IT

Dolores found other ways to supplement her income. After work, she baby-sat for several children, and on the weekends she and her husband provided party services for the community. She realized that when the welfare benefit ended, she would need to find a job and gain more education to earn a livable wage:

I got to get a job and a chance to get an education before I go out there looking for a job.

THEY CHOOSE THE SKILL FOR US

Wanting to read and write, Dolores looked for every opportunity to practice, including scheduled family literacy outings to the library with her child and grandchildren. I asked Dolores if she had the opportunity to practice reading and writing skills in her assigned activities at the nursing home. She replied,

The work skill is not reading or writing. They choose a skill for us. They going to put us in an activity, which I don't understand. Before I was in nursing. I lifted patients and I hurt my back. Lifting them without training, how can you lift them? They should train you before, like you should bend your knees before lifting, which I knew before. All you hear is that you were sent here to do the work.

We were told what to do and what not to do. Some minutes of your life, early in the morning there is nothing to do until Mom when everybody get changed. So you're not going to sit there and do nothing. The first thing they said is they going to write you up. You're not doing nothing.

So you feel like, let me give them a hand. This whole bed is a lot of work. We were doing their work while they were sitting down getting paid.

We used to feed them [residents], which I liked that. What we are doing now is exercising. I like to do things like that with them. They feel like their still alive. They want to do it. I don't like the part where your one on one with the resident. They want you to sit there with them. I want to be in a group where all of us could do something. Only one person? Why do I want to sit there and look at one person? They can hardly talk to me. There are a lot of residents that need me or can understand me. At first, they act like, "I don't want to be bothered."

IT'S IMPOSSIBLE TO START ON TIME

Dolores became the head workfare volunteer for the second-floor dayroom. She was responsible for setting up the dayroom for the day's activities, and the workfare volunteers assigned to the dayroom were under her authority. Cooperation with the nurses was essential in getting the program to start on time. If the nurses were short-staffed and residents were not ready, the volunteers had to wait. Dolores was concerned with how the volunteers were treated when the program was delayed, for they would be blamed for doing nothing.

It's impossible what she [Camilla] want. This morning, we came up to the dayroom. By the time all the rest of them was there, it's almost 11 o'clock. She's [Camilla] mad because the program's supposed to start at 10:30. But all the residents got in the dayroom at 11:00. What can we do? The nurse is telling us we can't bring them there earlier. We cannot do what Camilla said because this is what the nurse said. The nurse is responsible for the residents. Camilla's only responsible for the activity, not for the residents. Camilla came by the dayroom and said, "Where's Dolores?" and "Why are my programs not on?" I'm doing the transportation to the dayroom. She wants me to do it. I don't understand Camilla at all. We don't have enough time for the program because Camilla also wants us to be transporting people. What else she want us to do? Setting up. You setup the dayroom at 10:00 and they come in late. You only have 15 minutes to do the program. It's not going to work. The same thing with the movie. You see this movie here? Well, she changed the schedule to another activity, but if it was the movie today—let's say it starts at 2: 15—nobody is ready at 2:15. At 2:30, everybody is ready. Then at 2:30, they want the residents transported. You have until 3:00 to show the movie. What movie can you show in less than half an hour?

Dolores was frustrated. She saw the conflict between the nursing and activities departments but was unable to bring about any change because of the context of her consequence of her position in the hierarchy. She reflected on the meaning of work in the experience in the nursing home.

To me the meaning of work means, you know, like you willing to do or you want to do and not be forced to do. Like sometimes I come in and I'm ready to work. I know what my program is and I'm ready for this. And then all of a sudden everything changes. This don't mean nothing because she changes things around. So it's like you get depressed. You don't want to work.

Because if you get up early in the morning, you say, well, today I got to do arts and crafts, right? That's what you scheduled to do. That's what you know you do on Thursday or Friday. And then when you come here, you find out we not going to do that today. We going to change the schedule. Then why you make this for? Just like when you go to the doctor appointment. You are not going to change that appointment to someplace else unless it is an emergency. And you know you get depressions. She wants us to follow rules. Let us know ahead of time before that day gets here, so that week we prepare what's going to be. Don't let us come up here and fix everything for this program and then you go, "Oh no, no, no. I don't want this like this."

You know, sometimes I feel like saying a piece of my mind. And I don't want to go to her. So everybody gets depressed, upset with her—is getting stressed. They don't want to work. They don't feel like working. They here because they have to be here. Like we drafted. Just like when you go to army .You have to go. Not that you want to go. It is not good to work like that.

We can't do the program because she changes things. One second she say one thing. The next minute everything's changed. She need to put everything in writing for herself and make sure she know what she saying because it seems like she forget.

We work, but it's not the same like before. We used to love coming to work, and we felt good and we make the residents feel good. Now we got stress, and you not helping anybody if you're stressed. Because you doing the work just because you have to do it, not because it comes out of your heart.

Now she want us to help feed the residents. She made the biggest mistake she could make. She used to give us 15 minutes, right, that we used to go out and smoke a cigarette. Then we go for lunch. She got one day so angry at I don't know who that she said the 15 minutes is out of limit. She took it away from us. We used to go and smoke a cigarette, the 15 minute break, come back here and feed the residents. She took the break away from us and now all the girls are feeding nobody. That's it. So now nobody want to feed.

She gave us the break back thinking because she know she made a mistake, thinking we still going to feed them. We take our 15 minutes. We still don't want to feed the residents because she act like she—what you call a person that could demand, tell you what to do all the time?

We're here to do activity. That's not feeding people, okay. We don't have to do nothing but just activity. Activity don't have nothing to do with nursing, feeding, bathing, nothing like that. I told her, we ain't going to do no feeding, and we all going to get together whenever we feel like it is necessary.

The rest of the things we do. We don't make beds anymore. I did that for two years, and I helped them with the mop. Anyway, next year if I'm still in this program, I'm going to daycare. I'm getting tired of this. I want to deal with kids. This is too much.

Already feeling powerless to make any kind of changes within the environment, Dolores spoke to people in power when she was distressed about practices in the nursing home that she considered wrong.

And without using my name, there's been investigation. And it changed a lot. I seen it change a lot from when I first came here. I know what's right and what's wrong. I don't care what they tell me. If I see something wrong, it is wrong. I didn't tell them because at first I did tell them and they said like, "Watch what you're doing. Don't work this way. You going to work the other way." So I went the other way that wouldn't involve me. But I was involved, and I see a lot of change. It's like when you know you do something right that you helped them.

Shortly after this interview, Dolores left the nursing home in anger after a dispute because she felt she had been wrongfully accused of something. Later, during a phone conversation, she told me that she did not want to chance losing her temper and ending up in jail again. Taking control of the situation, she asked for another workfare assignment and was transferred to a community soup kitchen. Her absence had a profound effect on the volunteers, for they had lost an imaginative and energetic leader and peer.

BETTY: THIS HERE IS MY DREAM

Betty was a single mother of seven children. When we met, her 20-year-old son had just been arrested for a suicide attempt. His drug abuse, along with mental health and other cognitive issues, placed much strain on the family's sense of physical and emotional safety. Betty had begun her assignment at the nursing home two years earlier while living in a shelter. Her husband had been incarcerated and deported, leaving the family without money to pay the mortgage, so Betty had taken her children to a shelter, where they remained until she obtained Section 8 housing.

Getting to work on time was a problem for Betty. It took her two hours to travel to the nursing home. In addition, two younger daughters were in and out of the hospital for congenital hip disorders, and Betty had to take them to their medical appointments. Her adolescent daughter refused to go to school, and Betty was conflicted about leaving her home alone, but if Betty stayed home, she would lose her benefit. On the other hand, if she did not get the girl to school, the Bureau of Child Welfare would open her case and take away her children. Ironically, coming to work at the nursing home provided Betty relief from her family problems, but yet she perceived inequity in the workfare situation. When she reflected on her need for time off to take care of her children or go for a week to visit her husband, she was trapped by the program's inflexibility, as she had no other means of support:

> *If you had your own job, you could take days, but not on welfare. You don't get no sick days, no leave out, no vacation. You have to work. If you don't work, you get nothing, you know.*

Betty was also coping with some medical problems of her own. Diagnosed with high cholesterol, she had been told she must change her diet to prevent a stroke. In addition, she was having shoulder pains in her shoulder and, overall, feared taking medication. Her doctor advised her to exercise to gain control over her condition. She talked about how to fit in exercise with her work schedule and family responsibilities:

> *When I get home, I feel tired, like you ready to go to bed. I could do like about an hour or half an hour. You know, like move your legs and stuff like that for half an hour. Once you get into the habit, it then comes like nothing.*

LITERACY

Betty perceived her lack of education to be her greatest barrier. When she left school in the tenth grade to care for her younger siblings, she had been in a special education program. Still struggling to obtain basic skills, she found the opportunity to get an education as precious:

> *I have to go to school on Monday. The school is nice. I like it. The teacher is Mr. James. He is real nice. Right. And he tells you to read. I wish I had my poem. It was real nice about the people who are on welfare and how they feel about being on welfare. He got the book of people on welfare, and they write little poems and stuff. He takes them and put them in the book and stuff, and the next class that comes in can read it. So nice. I love it, too. Then you have only two days of school anyway. That's all, if you want to go back to school. Anyway, I got to go to school.*
>
> *I try to tell my kids that sometimes it can be a hassle when you know you see something and you know you can't read it and that bothers you. You see other people, and you say, "I wish," you know, "to get me a good job." You know, it makes you feel depressed sometimes, especially when you got kids, especially when you are struggling by yourself I have been struggling all my life by myself, so I know what it is like.*
>
> *I come here. I feel good. When I be around the old people, I feel good. And when I am at home, I feel stressed 'cause I am doing it by myself and they making me stressed. Because my kids are the type of kids that when things go wrong, they blame me for it. You should have did this. You should have did that. I should have done what I did the best I can do for you. What do you want me to do? I don't even know myself. Maybe keep my mind. I don't know.*

Betty found it very hard to separate her home life from her work experience. Her problems were so overwhelming and she felt so burdened that she could only describe in the interviews the details of her personal life. Her work experience was more pleasant, and she did not describe her activities with the residents. Her behavior suggested she was devoted to the residents to whom she was assigned, and they related to her emotionally.

DEVOTION TO RESIDENTS

The following playlet of Betty and Willa helping each other is an interaction I had observed and included in my field notes.

Actors: Willa (wheelchair-bound, alert nursing home resident)
           Three residents sitting around table with Willa
           Ida (nurse's aide)
           Andy (staff member)
           Esther (workfare volunteer)
           Betty (workfare volunteer)
           Connie (workfare volunteer)
           Boy (Connie's son)
           Ellen (researcher)
Setting: Second-floor dayroom at 11:00am

Against the far right wall, Betty sits with a group of residents around a large rectangular table. The residents are positioned in their wheelchairs next to each other, two residents on each side of the table. Three of the residents are cognitively impaired. Betty sits at the head of the table, adjacent to Willa, one of the four residents who is alert and oriented, with periods of confusion.

Betty is responsible for setting up an activity for the residents. She places plastic food items, such as hamburger and rolls, cheese, frankfurter, and roll, along with bright-colored connecting plastic forms, around the table within reach of each resident. The residents ignore the objects and stare into space.

Esther and I are observing the residents at the table with Betty. Esther points out how bored they appear to be. We walk over to the table, and I take a seat between Willa and Betty. I ask Willa, who knows me from my previous role as a therapist at the nursing home, if she knows Betty. This question leads to talk that gets Willa a lot of attention. Ida, a nurse's aide who was passing through the dayroom, begins a dialogue with Willa, teasing her about who had whose man. Willa puts Ida down.

Willa: *You're too old for James. He has a younger woman.*
Ida: (going along with it) *That's because I have the tailor. [her husband]*

During this interchange, Andy, a staff member from another department, comes around the table. He and Ida are standing together across the table from Willa.

Andy: (Opens his shirt) *Willa, look. I'm blowing my chest. Blow on my chest for me. (He walks around the table, picks up a frankfurter). Willa here's a frankfurter. (He proceeds to put the frankfurter in the roll. He stands next to her and blows on his chest.)*

Everyone is laughing. Willa seems to be taking this all in stride and questions the staff when their ideas sound illogical. Connie enters the room with her six-year old son. (She has a medical appointment with him later in the day and brought him to work with her to save time). They join this loud, raucous group.

Esther: *Andy, stop the chest blowing. We have children here.*

The crowd dissipates. Willa continues to talk.

Willa: *I still get my period.*
Betty: *You are too old to get your period, Willa.*
Willa: (Really angry) *I do, too!*
Betty: *You don't, Willa.* (making up a story). *I know this because I went into your room and spoke with the doctor.*
Willa: (Now very upset) *You did not!*
Esther: *Betty, please don't upset Willa*
Betty: (Correcting herself) *I'm sorry, Willa. I love you.*
Willa: *You don't love me. You don't love no one. You don't love yourself!*
Betty: (Tears coming into her eyes) *You know, that's just what I told my son the other day. I told him, "You don't love yourself." No one shoots themselves can love themselves.* (in a low voice) *He can't love himself.*

Willa: (calmer than before, she is quiet and looks at Betty, then takes her hand)

The above playlet illustrates that Betty did not know how to engage the residents with the materials she had found, nor did she know what to expect. She used her knowledge from past experiences observing residents in therapy and tried to simulate an experience. The volunteers were not trained how to choose an activity. In some instances, they had the freedom to try whatever activity they wanted, but at other times, they had to adhere to the activity schedule. Although Betty lacked experience, she attempted to do the right thing, and she used her interpersonal skills to connect with the residents as best she could. Willa forgave Betty for her teasing and then gave her the empathy of a friend.

THE INTERVIEW GIVES HOPE

In the spring, the volunteers were told about an interview for a nurse's aide position. Betty was quite excited about interviewing for the position. On the Friday before the interview, she sat with me in the dayroom and asked me to conduct a mock interview. She talked about what she would wear and how she would sit. When I returned the following week, Betty was upset, for the program was not going to approve the training required for the position.

I went on the interview that Monday right. We had to do the paper. She explained and asked us questions about our experience about old people and stuff like that. I showed her my certificate and my references. Okay, she did copies and she talked with us for a little while. Then she told us she was going to call us as to what day we are going to go for the interview. So she called us. She told us to call her the next day. So we called her, and she gave us an appointment the next day and stuff like that. We did the paper work and the tax stuff, all like that, right. Everything was dandy and stuff until I got back to school. Okay, I didn't ask questions. It just came up. They was asking us about the coffee. The coordinator said if anybody going to school for a home attendant, you can't go. They not paying baby-sitting money. You might not get carfare or baby-sitting money. I figure we can go on our own time. Whatever time we get. I guess the weekends, they don't have weekend classes. I guess the only thing we going to get is two days school and the job here.

They might do it or they might not. They said that they will, but sometimes things change.

TIGHTENING UP

In the past, Camilla and Dorothea did whatever they could to help the volunteers take advantage of outside training. However, over that year, the welfare-to-work program came under much attention and Camilla had to open her records to the program auditors. Any adjustments she made in work schedules for the volunteers was now under the scrutiny of the auditors, which had an impact upon the day-to-day flexibility the volunteers had once enjoyed.

You don't know when a person is going to do inspections and who is not there. They might call us one by one. That is what Dorothea is afraid of 'cause they doing a lot of specials. A lot of people come and they go. So they try to keep to themselves. If I can take it, I will take the training, but I don't know. It's no guarantee.

Betty was referring to home-attendant work. It would be risky to give up her welfare benefit for unsteady work that also had no benefits. However, getting a private case in addition to receiving welfare usually lasted longer and paid more. Betty's sister was employed that way.

My little sister works for an agency. You know, she have a certificate right? Well, my other sister, she only doing four hours, and that's only two weeks. You have to keep a patient two weeks. When two weeks is up, there is no guarantee that you will have another patient for the next two weeks. They cut into her check for that and your food stamps. What saves her is that she got a private case. She used to work with the lady on the two weeks, and then the lady couldn't afford to deal with the agency no more. Then the family wanted a private case, so the family asked her, because they know her, and that is how she came to get the private case in the evening. If she didn't do the class and then work the two weeks for the lady, she would never have that. It's worth it to get a private case. Trust me, it is good to have. I like working with old people. I really like it.

Betty was ambivalent about the opportunity to take the training if the program would be able to find a way to let them go. She feared that if she did any training activities outside of the daily program, the system would foul up her case, a fear based on other workfare volunteers' experiences, such as that of Florence.

> *I don't want them to mess up the roster paperwork. You understand what I mean? Sometimes things like that happen. That's why a few people working here is not here. Like Florence–you know Florence, the one who wore white. They messed up her roster and that is why she been home all this time. They messed up her baby-sitting money. Everybody thought she had a job, but she didn't. Things were hard for her. The baby-sitting money was helping her pay the bills. Her rent was behind $900 and everything. She had a hard time. It took her a couple of months. She had to borrow money and everything. That happened to a couple of peoples. I don't know what happened. They be doing something different. It happen to a lot of peoples.*

WHAT ARE YOU GOING TO DO?

Betty was discouraged about finding a job. Her time was coming to an end, and she had no plan in case she could not find a job. She knew she could never do anything illegal and, if necessary, would resort to begging.

> *If you don't find nothing by your time is up, you get cut off, and that is going to be the end of that. I be wondering how these peoples going to make it. After six months, if you don't find nothing, what are you going to do? They get completely cut off in six months. You don't get anything. I have seen that happen. They have a hard time making it. Your rent start backing up, your bills. That is what I am afraid of. I could get a job at the fast food restaurant, but that is not going to pay my bills. I can do without certain things, but what about the phone. My phone is for important business, and the lights you definitely need that. If you got no money, what are you going to do? Especially if you are a single mom with kids, it is very hard. They don't have enough jobs for everybody. People that don't have no skill or education, what are they going to do, sleep in the streets? I think that looks like that is going to happen to me.*
> *That is what is going to happen. They are going to start killing each other. They want money to feed their kids. They maybe a single*

parent. They have to feed their kids. They just there without an ed-
ucation. A lot of people out here like that, you know. They have no
skill, no high school diploma. You understand me, they take what
they can get if they can get it. A lot of mens live off their women. I
see that all the time. Can't depend on no man. l have no help with
my bills. I go do what I got to do. That's that. But I wish I could
come off, but I know that I am not going to do no better. It is too
late.

You have to have money to get where you going, and if they cut
me off, I will be too busy trying to feed my kids. If I got cut off, I
won't have a place to live, that's for sure. I got to eat. I don't know
what I would do. I never thought about it. I don't know. I would not
sell my body. I wouldn't steal from nobody. I would ask if l had to. I
would go on the train and beg. There are a lot of people out there
who are doing that. It isn't just me. When they cut me off, there is
going to be a lot of them cut off–about 2, 000. They got on the same
time I did, so I won't be feeling too bad (laughing) but I will be cry-
ing everyday. Where my next dollar coming from or a loaf of
bread, I don't know.

When summer arrived, Esther helped Betty get her a job at the amusement park for several weeks. Their friendship that had developed at the
nursing home helped each of them to cope with great difficulties in their
family life. Betty was convinced that if she only had the intelligence of an
educated person, she would be able to get a job. By the end of the year, she
was reading short stories and shared one with me. Despite her fatalistic attitude, she kept trying every day.

REFLECTIONS ON PARTICIPANTS' RECOMMENDATIONS

In each workfare experience narrative, the participant, based on her
daily experience in the program, contributes her perspective on how the
workfare program can be improved through policy changes and program
implementation. The recommendations for change expressed by the participants fall under five categories: Work Ethics, Professional Development, Work Skills, Work Policies, and Education. Every participant
made some recommendations for at least some of the categories; sometimes these recommendations were stated directly, but other times they
were suggestions that came from their stories. Table 1 illustrates these
recommendations.

While the participants often discussed their perspectives with one another, their ideas remained within the group. They felt very strongly about their suggestions and gave me, as the researcher, an opportunity to organize their ideas with the hope that other women might benefit from their experience. Four years later, Peterson (2002) addresses several of the recommendations suggested by the participants of this study. Issues of racial/ethnic disparity and welfare-to-work strategies raised by the volunteers and validated by Peterson continue to be part of the ongoing welfare-reform debate. The voices of the participants and other TANF mothers need to be part of the conversation that shapes policy; they have first-hand experience and can contribute to the process of improving lives for poor mothers and their families.

doi:10.1300/J004v23n03_07

TABLE 1. Participant Recommendations for Change in Workfare Program

	Florence	Agnes	Connie	Esther	Dolores	Betty
Work Ethic	Give choice in work assignment. Sensitivity to immigrants. Acknowledge fear of racial, ethnic, age discrimination		Acknowledge Fear of racial, ethnic, age Discrimination		Advocate for quality and humane resident care.	
Professional Development	Identify needs of women working for first time.		Reinforce Successful Performance with respect. Provide Opportunities to help Volunteers grow and develop skills.	Reinforce Successful Performance with respect.		Plan for transition to employment
Work Skills			Provide Newcomers With experienced volunteers' Tips for Success		Train volunteers to work with residents	
Work Policies	Consistency in workfare assignments.	Transform workfare into paid employment				Give work benefits, vacations, sick *days*.
Education	Enhanced literacy and special training programs. Paid certified nursing asst. program during workfare hrs.	Enhanced literacy and special training programs. Paid certified nursing asst. program during workfare hrs.	Enhanced literacy and special training programs.	Enhanced literacy and special training programs. Full-time education vs. workfare assignments		Enhanced literacy and special training programs

Chapter 8

Insecurity:
Issues and Concerns

SUMMARY. I present the volunteers' issues and concerns in their own words, including their insecurity about food and homelessness. In this chapter, I address the impact these problems had on their children's lives. doi:10.1300/J004v23n03_08 *[Article copies available for a fee from The Haworth Document Delivery Service: 1-800-HAWORTH. E-mail address: <docdelivery@haworthpress.com> Website: <http://www.HaworthPress. com> © 2007 by The Haworth Press, Inc. All rights reserved.]*

KEYWORDS. Homelessness, food insecurity, BCW, resiliency

INTRODUCTION

The volunteers often spoke of how they were afraid of losing control of necessary resources for survival; homelessness and hunger were primary fears. They knew that if they could not provide a stable home, they were in danger of losing their children to BCW. Some already had an open Bureau

[Haworth co-indexing entry note]: "Insecurity: Issues and Concerns." Greer, Ellen. Co-published simultaneously in *Occupational Therapy in Mental Health* (The Haworth Press, Inc.) Vol. 23, No. 3/4, 2007, pp. 127-132; and: *Women's Immersion in a Workfare Program: Emerging Challenges for Occupational Therapists* (Ellen Greer) The Haworth Press, 2007, pp.127-132. Single or multiple copies of this article are available for a fee from The Haworth Document Delivery Service [1-800-HAWORTH, 9:00 a.m. - 5:00 p.m. (EST). E-mail address: docdelivery@haworthpress.com].

of Child Welfare (BCW) case, which subjected them to ongoing surveillance. Given the inconsistent system, the volunteers were often financially and emotionally on the edge. The system frequently made mistakes that placed the families in jeopardy of food insecurity and loss of shelter. Attempting to keep things together was sometimes overwhelming. As mothers, they were in need of assistance from many levels of support that did not exist.

IN THEIR OWN WORDS

Betty did not feel safe in her home.

Here in my new home, not so comfortable. Feel a little bit safe, not much, because the place is not what I thought it was going to be.

Multiple environmental and emotional problems led to her uncomfortable feelings. Coming from a shelter, she had wanted an apartment that was not falling apart, but this landlord had not taken care of the apartment–paint was peeling, the ceiling was falling down, and mice were running rampant. If she had not taken this apartment, she would have remained homeless with her seven children. Once she became settled, her older son's drug activity created a chaotic and dangerous atmosphere in their home life. Betty was scared. Connie, unlike Betty, felt safe in her home. She lived in an apartment building where neighbors looked out for one another. Her greatest concern was not having the money from welfare to pay the rent or buy food for the children. At times, the welfare system had missed payments for rent and food, leading to crisis situations for Connie's family. She had been threatened by eviction, and her children had been hungry. Connie coped by turning toward her faith, as well asking her mother for help.

If you don't work, you lose your benefit, and that means homelessness. I don't want to be in that situation. You understand there were times when like the rent, I was caught, and the landlord was telling me that he was going to evict me cause public assistance hasn't paid the rent. So I called the Lord, "I don't think I am going to make it." I need an apartment. I am there because I can't afford a new thing for the time being. You can't be afraid. Your kids are hungry and they say, "Mommy, I am hungry." You have to do something. I have been there. You open the refrigerator and there is not food. What do I do? I don't panic. I call my mother.

"Do you have any food or do you have money?" "If I don't have the money, I will get it for you." If not for that, a lot of people don't have that. It is not my mother's responsibility. It is mine. I will get it if I got to clean your house to make sure my son eat.

The neighbors in Connie's building looked out for her and her children.

There are times I don't have food because the food stamps they give isn't enough, but my neighbors always know, and knock. "This is for your children. This is for you." One day I didn't cook. I was sick with my stomach, and I was in bed. They took care of me even though I was in bed. They took care of me. Like yesterday, I was home and they came and took care of me. That is why I say, if I move, I don't know. Everybody in the building is very close.

Connie's problem was more complex than just mistakes in the welfare system. She stated that there was not enough in the food stamp benefit that she received. Although her mother said that she would try to find the money for her, Connie said, *"I can't bother my mother, she has bills too, and I don't have friends that have that kind of money."* Understandably, Connie did not want to move from her apartment. With supports so fragile, her neighbors may have been a lifeline for her when she was without money or food. Connie was resilient, having learned not to panic, not to be afraid in face of threats, and to take responsibility to do whatever necessary to feed her family.

Florence had a similar ethic about taking responsibility for oneself in face of the threat of homelessness. Living with her aunt, she had a safe home environment for her children, and her welfare benefit paid for her half of the rent. Her childhood history of being homeless and abandoned by her father heightened the importance she placed on self-sufficiency.

I am not getting financial support. I think even if you have a husband, you have to live your life in a sense that if the person can't be around tomorrow you can cope. That is why I am looking for a job that I know I won't end up homeless or something I could manage until I come off public assistance.

Florence could not rely on her children's father for material support because he was in another country. She made it clear that family and friends could support her emotionally but they were not a resource to put food on the table. Like Connie, Florence had a strong faith and a mother who tried to help her.

> *In the long run, it is only family and whatever. If you have friends that are real close like family, they will be there for you physically, but they are not going to pay your rent for you, and they are not going to put food on the table for you. There are some things you have to do for yourself. My mother is there if the children need anything. If it wasn't for her, I don't think my children would have clothes.*

Florence accepted that she needed to rely on herself to provide for her children. However, the admission that her children would not have clothes if it were not for her mother was another indication that the welfare benefit was not enough to provide for basic needs.

Agnes was living in a two-family house, supported by a Section 8 housing benefit. Maintaining the home was problematic, for the first-floor tenants did not keep the hallways that led to Agnes's apartment clean. Most distressing for Agnes was the news that the house was being put up for sale and she was in danger of losing her apartment: *"It is up to the new landlord if he wants Section 8 because some don't want it. If the new people buy the house, if they accept Section 8, I can stay there and I won't have to move."* In her resilient manner, she protected her family against homelessness by having a plan and implementing a search to find a new Section 8 home, should she find herself on the street.

Another example of resiliency in protecting one's family from homelessness was Dolores's solution of starting a micro-enterprise in her home.

She and her husband had become known for their baked party cakes and over time had received catering orders from their community. Dolores had arranged to maintain the house in which they lived and, as supers of the house living in the basement apartment, they managed with the small welfare stipend.

Esther had been homeless when she graduated from drug rehabilitation. Although before that time she had lived in her mother's apartment her entire life, she lost the apartment after her mother died because she had been incarcerated for drug abuse. Housing projects can evict tenants under such conditions. Esther knew she was to be reunited with her children and needed a home. She found a lawyer who fought for her and won back the rights to her apartment.

REFLECTIONS ON THREATS TO SECURITY

While all participants were insecure about food and homelessness, some had taken proactive steps to keep that circumstance at a distance.

Other participants had said they would take responsibility and do whatever was necessary, but they had not taken any actual steps to prepare for the possibility of homelessness or to appeal for more food stamps to remove hunger from daily life. What is unique is the relationship between each participant's response to insecurity about food and shelter and the continual threat of losing her children to the Bureau of Child Welfare (BCW). Basically, participants' responses to insecurity could be put into the following seven categories: autonomy, community, faith, family, pro-action, collaboration, and legal representation.

Betty's response falls under the first category, autonomy. She was in crisis, living daily with the threat of violence in her home but did not believe she could reach out to anyone to change her situation. Instead, she relied on her own resources and strategies to maintain some kind of equilibrium–although she had come to realize she could no longer control her life situation.

In contrast, Connie's issues with food insecurity were assuaged by a caring community. Her neighbors were aware of her situation, and she welcomed their assistance. Similarly, Dolores had set up a micro-enterprise and established relations with her community so that her neighbors would seek out her catering services. Florence's and Betty's response to insecurity focused on their faith in God. When food, housing, and financial insecurities became threatening, they turned to their own spiritual resource, asking God for help. Florence also counted on her family for emotional support in times of food and financial insecurity. Although her family could not provide the money to cover the rent when Florence was no longer in the system, her mother did provide clothing for the children, thus alleviating some distress.

Agnes and Dolores both proactively took control of their insecure situations through independently implementing a plan to prepare for the future. Agnes began looking for a new home before possibly being evicted. Dolores began developing a business so that when she was finished with welfare, she would have the financial resources to survive.

Dolores also used collaboration to respond to insecurity. She saw the benefit in working together with her husband to secure their livelihood in the face of welfare ending. She recognized her own limitations and saw how her husband's strengths and talents complemented her own capability. With this fusion of talents and cooperation, Dolores demonstrated how collaboration in a relationship can enhance the potential for survival in face of insecurity of food, shelter, and finances.

Finally, Esther used legal assistance as a response. Because of her drug history, she had to fight to gain security of shelter. She was aware of her powerlessness within the system and turned to legal representation to fight for her. Winning back her rights both to her home and children, Esther learned that responding to insecurity must sometimes go beyond one's own resources, that one may have to turn to the principles of democracy and social justice.

doi:10.1300/J004v23n03_08

Chapter 9

Impact on the Children:
Problems and Solutions

SUMMARY. In this chapter, I examine the specific problem Betty had with her children because, in many ways, it represents the problems most of the volunteers had with their children. Her problem was the most extreme among the participants, and she involved the other volunteers in helping her look for a solution. The vignette that follows comes from my field logs, and it is followed with a layered response from Betty's peers. The vignette offers a close look at Betty's problems with her daughters and the dilemma she experienced in relation to coming to work when her children needed her. Betty told her story to Esther, Dolores, and me one morning in the dayroom. doi:10.1300/J004v23n03_09 *[Article copies available for a fee from The Haworth Document Delivery Service: 1-800- HAWORTH. E-mail address: <docdelivery@haworthpress.com> Website: <http://www.HaworthPress.com> © 2007 by The Haworth Press, Inc. All rights reserved.]*

KEYWORDS. Adversity, family disruption, risk factors, protective factors

[Haworth co-indexing entry note]: "Impact on the Children: Problems and Solutions." Greer, Ellen. Co-published simultaneously in *Occupational Therapy in Mental Health* (The Haworth Press, Inc.) Vol. 23, No. 3/4, 2007, pp. 133-141; and: *Women's Immersion in a Workfare Program: Emerging Challenges for Occupational Therapists* (Ellen Greer) The Haworth Press, 2007, pp. 133-141. Single or multiple copies of this article are available for a fee from The Haworth Document Delivery Service [1-800-HAWORTH, 9:00 a.m. - 5:00 p.m. (EST). E-mail address: docdelivery@haworthpress.com].

Available online at http://otmh.haworthpress.com
© 2007 by The Haworth Press, Inc. All rights reserved.
doi:10.1300/J004v23n03_09

INTRODUCTION

At least one child in each participant's family was experiencing serious problems. The nature of the problems differed among the families, ranging from poor school performance, behavioral problems, medical problems, school avoidance, dropping out, drug involvement, suicidal enactments, and incarceration. The one common thread was the distress the mothers reported over their children's falling behind in school, but each mother managed that distress differently. Most complained that when they returned home in the evenings, they were too tired to help their children with their homework. Although they did not have a conflict between work and mothering, they were overloaded by the long hours and labor in the nursing home and the multiple problems at home, including the multiple roles they played within their families.

BETTY'S DILEMMA

Betty wanted her children to finish high school. Her three oldest children had dropped out of high school, and the four youngest daughters, aged 7 to 14, were all having difficulties in school, with the youngest and the oldest at highest risk. Although the two middle girls had serious orthopedic problems, Betty never reported that they had problems in school. According to Betty, the seven-year-old had not passed even one test since she had started school. The 14-year-old simply refused to go to school.

Betty's 12-year-old daughter Katisha was recovering from hip surgery. Three of her daughters had been born with congenital hip problems that had become symptomatic at the time of adolescence. Increased weight gain precipitated the problem in all of the girls. Katisha had gained weight since they had moved into the new apartment. There was no recreational outlet for the girls in the neighborhood, so they stayed in the house after school and, as Betty said, ate "junk." When they had lived in the shelter in Manhattan, they had had a range of afternoon activities from which to choose, such as dance, gymnastics, and basketball. Now Betty did not want them to go outside because the neighborhood was not safe, so the girls occupied themselves with television and snacking.

On the Friday morning of this vignette, Betty explained that Katisha was in much pain from her recent surgery. Betty was frustrated because she wanted to be home to care for Katisha, but instead she has had to take Katisha to her oldest daughter, whom Betty does not trust will provide the proper care while Betty is at work.

Betty: *I couldn't stand looking at her limp anymore. I can't stand it, you hear? So I took her over to emergency. They took an X-ray and saw that she needed the surgery. The surgery came out good, but she has staples. My other daughter had the same surgery and she had stitches and healed, okay, but staples–she's gonna have a big scar.*

When I took her home, they gave her crutches. She has to learn to use them. It took us one hour to cross the street and walk down the block to my oldest daughter's house. But I'm worried because Katisha is crying. Her leg hurts, and I don't want her taking too much medication.

I hope my daughter doesn't keep giving it to her. It has codeine and that is addicting, isn't it? I can't be with her because I have to be here, but I don't know what I am going to do on Monday. I have no one to watch her. I don't have too many friends. My sons go out during the day to make money. You know what they doing!

Ellen: *Could their girlfriends baby-sit?*
Betty: *Their girlfriends are not the mother kind, you understand me? My daughter isn't, either.*

Betty took out the hospital papers to show us the history of Katisha's case. She also had a letter from Katisha's school. Betty needed to go to the school on Monday because Katisha had been absent for a month and Betty was worried that Katisha would fall behind in her work.

Ellen: *Can the school send a teacher to your home?*
Betty: *No one is there. How they going to send someone?*
Esther: [Becoming very upset, she is moving around in her chair] *They have to let you stay home with her. You can't leave her alone, or BCW is going to take your kids away.*
Betty: *I can't give a baby-sitter money 'cause I need the money, you understand me? And now I don't know what I'll do, 'cause they're going to be sending the baby-sitting money to the baby-sitter.*
Ellen: (I know how important the babysitting money has been to Betty, as she used it to buy clothing and other necessities for her children. She relied on the older children for childcare or left the girls alone after school until she got home.) *What will you do?*
Betty: *My friend will give it to me. They will send it to her and she will give it to me. You have to be ahead of these things and prepare*

>*for the changes or else you get nothing. I know what I am do-*
>*ing. Maybe I'll bring Katisha home with me this weekend. It*
>*hurts me when she be crying. I can't take it, but I don't want her*
>*taking that medication 'cause it might be dangerous.*

Just before lunch, Betty, Esther, and Dolores finished setting up the dayroom for the residents to have their lunch hour. The three of them were standing by the piano in the front of the dayroom, reviewing Betty's dilemma about having to leave her daughter on Monday and were not satisfied with the options available. Dolores crystallized the moral solution that had a problematic outcome for Betty.

Dolores: *Betty, you have to stay home with your daughter on Monday*
        and as long as she needs you, but if you don't show up here,
        you're gong to end up losing your babysitting money.

Esther, who recently regained custody of her children after many years, believed that to protect her relationship with her children, Betty needed to be proactive with the help of the other mothers in the same situation.

Esther: *Betty can't do this on her own. Come on. It's happening to all*
        of us. We women need to get together. We got to do something
        about this child-care problem for our teenagers.
        I just got mine back. There is no way when my son turns 13
        next month that I'm going to let him be alone in the house,
        especially with an open BCW case.
        But no one wants to get together. People are afraid. At
        school, there is a woman who is in charge of starting the un-
        ion. She has meetings with us, and we get together and talk
        about these things. This is not right. You have to come to the
        meeting.

Betty listened quietly. The three women walked out of the dayroom together to head for lunch. Esther and Dolores were in a deep discussion about the union meetings, and Betty drifted behind them. They walked toward the elevator, the door opened, and they went downstairs to check in at Camilla's office and then proceed to lunch.

During lunch in the cafeteria, I sat with Betty and Dolores. Esther had left to buy lunch in the neighborhood. Betty talked about her 14-year-old daughter, Shenae, who was not attending school, and Betty was concerned that she could not be home to supervise her.

Betty: *I need a therapist for Shenae, the 14-year-old. She won't go to school, and I don't know what to do. I'm not there. Every morning she wakes up, she comes out limping or some other problem. Every morning there is a physical problem and says she doesn't feel good.*

Dolores: (speaks strongly to Betty). *You got to go to BCW on Bradford Street before they come and take your kids away for doing nothing.*

Betty: *Dolores, I don't know where to go for help, but I don't want to go to BCW. I tried the PINS* [Persons in Need of Supervision], *went to court, but that didn't work. Nothing helps her.*

Dolores: (sternly) *You have an open BCW case. What's wrong with you, Betty? Go to them for advice. They'll end up taking your younger girls away because* of *your teenager.*

Betty: *My son needs counseling, too. He's already on the books as having something wrong with him. He shot himself. He's on crack. Maybe he can get SSI. He was in special ed, was always a little slow. He's his father's son, and his father was committed to the looney bin. I want therapy for all my girls, someone to sit down with them and talk with them.*

Dolores: (changes her tone, softer, tries to be helpful) *You know, counselors can come to the house.*

Betty: (nods in agreement) *Yeah, I remember when a counselor came to the house to talk with Shenae, and Shenae didn't say a word. She didn't cooperate. You know, if she likes the lady, she will talk. If she doesn't like the lady, all she'll say is, "Yeah, right."*

The mood around the table is hopeless. Dolores quits offering suggestions. Betty begins to talk about wanting to escape from the program.

Betty: *I just want to get out of this program. I want to get out of here. I don't want to be doing this, but I need a job.*

VOLUNTEERS' PERSPECTIVES

Betty's dilemma was shared with the other volunteers later in the day. Following are the perspectives of Agnes, Connie, and Florence regarding Betty's problem.

Agnes

Betty lost control over her girls! I tell my girls, "If you don't go to school and you not doing good, I'm coming to school with you and I'm gonna sit in your classroom until you learn what you got to learn." And they don't like that.

Like when my girls, Arlo, Tiffany, and Kim, all failed their report card this last time, I put them on punishment. No hitting. They can't watch television or go outside. I'm too tired at night and I can't help them, so they they got to study on their own. My youngest, Kim, she the smart one. She reads all day. I don't know why she failing. Tiffany, now she is all talking into people's business and getting into trouble. I tell people nobody is going to touch her 'cause I'll go straight to the mother and smack if I have to. She's failing 'cause she more interested in talking than studying. Arlo, she's my oldest. She was getting 70s, 80s. I told her that is okay, she's passing, but her father yells at her and says only 100% is good and nothing less. She's mad at her father, and I guess me too. I have a new boyfriend and things are different. They never see me with another man except their father. Their father—now he got a woman, and the girls see him in bed with her. I told his friend if she come into my house, I will pluck her. She better stay away from me.

I notice the girls acting funny, so I started a monthly meeting where they can say whatever they want, about me, their father, about boys. You should hear what they ask. I want them to learn how to express their feelings so they don't hold it in or get violent later. I'm just learning how to express my own feelings about my mother and father and their strictness and hitting.

Anyway, maybe Betty should try bringing her girls together herself and let them talk about what they feeling. If she needs time off, she always here, and them downstairs will help her out. They understand.

Connie

I know why Betty wants to get out of this program. All year here in the nursing home and we accomplished nothing, and we got problems at home. It's not easy to know what to do. Now I have an open BCW case just like Betty. My 12-year-old son Allen started having problems in school. He hit the teacher and they called me in. I went in on open school week. I met with all his teachers, and we worked as a team to come up with a plan to help Allen improve in his learning. He was failing some subjects. English is hard for him. We speak Spanish at home, and we have heavy accent.

But my son hurt me. He told the school I am not feeding him, and they reported me. So now I have to take him for therapy. I'm too tired at the end of the day, and I have to go pick up my little one. So we missed some appointments.

At night I sit with him. We go over our words, we work on our accent, and we follow the teacher's plan. He starting to do better. My other son, he is afraid of his prosthetic arm. I got to sit with him. I tell him if he is afraid and don't practice with the arm, he won't be able to take care of himself and do what the other boys do. It's not easy 'cause he's disabled and dressing him in the morning and undressing him at night takes a long time.

You got to work as a team. Betty needs to meet with her girl's teachers, get a plan, and then sit with them at night. Until her daughter is better, she got to get permission to stay home with her.

Florence

Betty works here every day. Sometimes I see she brings her children with her. I wonder why they aren't in school. She's got lots of medical appointments. You can't be everywhere at once. If she took the girls back to school, she wouldn't be able to come to work.

There must be a way for Betty to appeal so she can stay home with her daughters. She has a crisis, and that can make you bug out. I know how she feels. Every morning I get aggravation from my 10-year-old son. He is slow, always forgets stuff, and we end up missing his bus. Then I have to take him to school, and I might be late for work.

My son John is being taken out of the gifted class. He has a bad temper, and he's not doing his work. He follows the boys who get in trouble. I worry he'll end up like my brother. He drove us crazy. He was into drugs and has been homeless. John is like his father, too. His father had a temper. John is "sometimish." What I mean is that sometimes he does good, but then he sometimes he fights too hard with his sisters. I talk to him and explain how he needs to do good in school and grow up to be a good man. I tell him if he's not acting good, he can end up in the streets, like the homeless we see.

I don't know how we're going to help these kids when we're so worried if we have enough money. We're so tired, our eyes are closing when we get home.

DILEMMA IS RESOLVED

The following week, Betty stayed home with her daughter on Monday. She arranged to have her friend whom she trusted stay with Katisha.

Although she felt powerless to help Shenae and her older sons, she was determined to save the younger children before BCW might get a hold of them. She began to talk about sending the young girls to live with their father in the Caribbean. She needed to begin planning how to protect the younger children from the older ones.

REFLECTIONS ON SUGGESTED STRATEGIES

The volunteers had different perspectives on how to manage Betty's dilemma, and their individual strategies stemmed from what had worked for them. Dolores had learned how to get help from the authorities, to get them on her side, so she had suggested that Betty go to BCW. However, Betty knew this was a dangerous proposition, that if BCW became aware of the problems with her older sons, she was sure to lose her girls. Having to hide this problem was isolating for Betty.

Esther suggested Betty take a pro-active stance. Experienced in standing up for her rights, she saw it as a powerful move to gather other women together and talk about the problem of child care that was affecting all of them in one way or another. That was a good suggestion, but Betty was uncomfortable speaking out in a group about social justice issues. She also wanted to maintain some degree of privacy regarding the volatility of what was occurring in her home.

Agnes's style was to take leadership to solve problems, and she had suggested Betty meet with her girls in a group. Betty may have been able to do this if she had not always felt undermined by her older children.

Connie's suggestion to get help from the teachers was founded in her philosophy that working as a team brings success. Betty, challenged with literacy issues and just learning to read, was not at a point in her own education where she could help her daughters with their school work. Her focus at home was to provide a clean environment, food, and other basic necessities.

Florence had suggested that Betty appeal her situation so that she could stay home for a period of time with her daughter. Florence was not afraid to tackle the system, but Betty was, fearing doing anything that would mess up the roster.

All these solutions had merit but also presented possible roadblocks. In her resilient way, Betty found a way to get her friend to care for her daughter and, at the same time, finally accepted the reality of her home life. It was possible that she would have to send her children away to their father to keep them safe and yet within the family.

Although it is not clear exactly why the participants' children were failing, perhaps the impact of their mothers' fatigue and distress with the overload of family and work responsibilities may have diminished the mother's energy to provide the unique attention and assistance that each child required. Not all the children were failing, but only Florence's two daughters were doing well. Although Florence faced a financial crisis, she was surrounded by family supports. Her family of professional nurses was involved in providing for the needs of her children, and, in that way, her case stood apart from that of the other volunteers.

doi:10.1300/J004v23n03_09

Chapter 10

Despite False Hopes,
Forced Transition Creates Growth

SUMMARY. In this chapter, I discuss how each of six stages applied to the reported experiences of the volunteers, drawing examples from field logs and interviews and the data reflected in the previous chapters. doi:10.1300/J004v23n03_10 *[Article copies available for a fee from The Haworth Document Delivery Service: 1-800- HAWORTH. E-mail address: <docdelivery@haworthpress.com> Website: <http://www.HaworthPress.com> © 2007 by The Haworth Press, Inc. All rights reserved.]*

KEYWORDS. Compliance, engagement, conflict, family and work spillover, dynamic process, struggle, contemplation

INTRODUCTION

Studies focusing on how welfare reform since 1996 has affected women in poverty have found that the transition from welfare to work led to either

[Haworth co-indexing entry note]: "Despite False Hopes, Forced Transition Creates Growth." Greer, Ellen. Co-published simultaneously in *Occupational Therapy in Mental Health* (The Haworth Press, Inc.) Vol. 23, No. 3/4, 2007, pp. 143-152; and: *Women's Immersion in a Workfare Program: Emerging Challenges for Occupational Therapists* (Ellen Greer) The Haworth Press, 2007, pp. 143-152. Single or multiple copies of this article are available for a fee from The Haworth Document Delivery Service [1-800-HAWORTH, 9:00 a.m. - 5:00 p.m. (EST). E-mail address: docdelivery@haworthpress.com].

low-wage work or to no work (Beckman, 2002; Maine Equal Justice Project, 2002) Community Service Society, 1999). These studies have also found that a significant number of families have experienced food and housing insecurity and homelessness after leaving the TANF program.

Similarly, the nursing home volunteers in this study noted that the program itself did not lead to work, and food and housing insecurity and parenting children were dominant issues and concerns (see Chapters 8 and 9). The data suggests that when one moved from the welfare-recipient role into the new role of workfare volunteer, common thematic patterns emerged. Their transition was not linear; instead, they went through a dynamic process when making the transition into the new workfare volunteer role. I believe that the volunteers in the mandated work program experienced the following six thematic lived aspects of forced transition: (1) compliance; (2) engagement in work activities; (3) conflict with authority; (4) family-work spillover; (5) struggling with the system; and (6) contemplating change.

STAGE 1: COMPLIANCE WITH PROGRAM RULES

Complying with the program rules refers to the volunteer following the formal guidelines for entering the program. This included attending orientation, interviewing for a work-activity assignment, accepting the role of volunteer in the nursing home, and cooperating with the work behavior rules. For each volunteer in this study, compliance was a unique process; although all had complied, their reactions and attitudes towards compliance were diverse.

Both Connie and Florence had been anxious about entering the program. They had wondered whether they would be able to do the work and whether they would be rejected because of race and ethnicity. But whereas Florence had a positive attitude, Connie had a negative attitude. Florence stated, *"This program offers me the opportunity to prepare for my field in nursing,"* while Connie said, *"At the beginning I had a nasty attitude because I was forced to be here."*

At first, Dolores had not wanted to be in the program; instead, she wanted to be home with her son. Only after two years of compliance did she see any value to the program. On the other hand, Betty found it easy to comply. She viewed the program as her *"bread and water"*; the nursing home was a safe haven, and the baby-sitting money helped her provide clothing for her daughters. Agnes complied with a goal in mind: to learn skills, get training, obtain her degree, and move on with her life. Esther complied but viewed the program as a waste of time.

STAGE 2: ENGAGEMENT IN WORK ACTIVITIES

Engagement in work activities refers to the active process of purposeful doing and learning within the nursing home setting. Being engaged in work activities with the nursing home residents and staff led the volunteers to become aware of their unique capabilities. The volunteers had not known the capabilities that emerged through the engagement in work activities beforehand. In some ways, this stage was a form of self-discovery.

In working with her patient Alice, Agnes learned that she had the capacity to comfort, to provide love and attention, and to be empathetic. She also learned that she was capable of furthering her education. She obtained her GED during her workfare assignment and said that she would consider college once she obtained a job.

Florence was challenged by disrespectful staff members, and she found she could be verbally attacked and still respond constructively. She was proud that she could work with all kinds of people. In working with the residents, she learned that she could make mistakes when making assumptions and that she was capable of correcting those mistakes. Empathy was a newfound interpersonal skill, as she put herself in the place of the residents.

Connie became aware of her capability to help her peers by sharing her own experiences. She also found that she could help the residents assigned to her by being sensitive to their needs. *"I have learned how to be with residents."* Visiting the residents daily, she read to them, talked to them, and formed relationships.

Although Esther was the most negative about working with the residents, she was cooperative and loyal. Feeding the residents and helping her peers when they needed assistance or company taught her that she was capable of giving. She was the only participant who discovered she was capable of being directly proactive and fighting for fairness. As Esther told Betty in response to Betty's dilemma (see Chapter 8), *"This is happening to all of us. We have to talk about this situation."* She informed Betty that there was a woman from the union at school who was meeting with the women. Although Esther was quiet, she was finding her voice.

Dolores found her ability to lead her peers and to advocate for the residents. She was the linchpin that held the second-floor volunteers together. She helped her peers by covering for them when they could not arrive at the site on time, particularly Betty, who was often late because of her daughters' medical appointments. Dolores's kindness was returned with her peers' loyalty and affection. Dolores also learned that some authorities could not be dealt with directly. She discovered that events or occurrences that she believed wrong or needed changing could only be dealt with by going underground. In her own way, she made various changes in the care of the residents, and this gave her great satisfaction.

Betty found that she was good at caring for the elderly. She was kind and loyal. Literacy was a barrier, but as the year progressed, she found that she was capable of reading and writing.

STAGE 3: CONFLICT WITH AUTHORITY

Conflict with authority was a stressful experience for the volunteers. They had to address their own attitudes toward authority within a hierarchy, as well as among peers. Issues of stigma, marginalization, and demeaning staff comments were painful to tolerate. Underlying the problems with conflict with authority were the volunteers' past negative experiences, along with their need for respect and recognition for the work they were doing at the nursing home.

Esther's perceptions of Camilla's demoralizing treatment of the volunteers in Chapter 7 vividly illustrates how painful she found this stage. Esther struggled with Camilla's judgments about how the volunteers spent their money. She felt persistently stigmatized by Camilla's comments regarding the values of poor women.

Dolores's conflict with authority centered around her frustration with Camilla's changing the program schedule. However, she could not verbalize the anger she felt with Camilla, making her feel depressed and being forced to work. She compared it to being drafted into the armed forces, a soldier who must obey authority. Because Dolores was a leader, she was able to gather the volunteers together and develop a plan against the authority. When a smoking break had been taken away, she convinced the group to resist and take power against Camilla by not feeding the residents. Ultimately, Dolores's conflict with authority led to her leaving the facility when accused of taking her own records. Dolores was so enraged, but rather than express her hurt and frustration, she left for another site.

Interestingly, except for Dolores, no volunteer was accepted as a leader, and when Dolores left the nursing home, the volunteers formed a system of teamwork so that no single person was giving orders. Whenever Camilla assigned a volunteer to lead an activity, their "you're not my boss" attitude created conflict. To avoid this dynamic, the focus of teamwork served to keep everyone equal and protected them when authorities such as Camilla and Dorothea came upstairs to observe their job performance.

Betty and Florence had the least problems with conflict. Betty was easygoing and street smart. She knew how to take care of herself and to get what she needed from the authority. For example, she had wanted to travel to the Caribbean to visit her husband. Her son had recently made a suicide attempt and she was under great strain. However, leaving the site would jeopardize her benefit. Having explained her problem to Dorothea, the Activities Supervisor, she resolved the problem and was covered for the week.

Agnes worked by herself and followed the rules, but she would become enraged when volunteers were blamed for someone else's misconduct. Whenever a meeting would be called to address the latest misconduct, such as forged time sheets, her temper would flare; she would throw a chair and complain loudly to her peers, rather than express the unfairness of this practice to Camilla and Dorothea.

Connie was the only volunteer who wanted to work out her feeling of conflict regarding Camilla. When she returned to the nursing home after her reassessment–which occurs after a workfare cycle is completed–she did not get along with Camilla, so she asked if she could speak with her privately. During that meeting, Connie told her, "*When you are upset with me I want you to talk with me in private. I want to be respected. Do not yell at me in front of others.*"

Connie continued to tell Camilla what she expected of her, and, over time, they resolved their problematic relationship. When I left the nursing home, Camilla told me that she felt Connie had the most potential among the volunteers to be employed.

STAGE 4: FAMILY AND WORK SPILLOVER

Family and work spillover refers to the interrelationship between home and work problems that could not be contained within either context. In most cases, the spillover appeared to occur in the home-to-work direction. Volunteers were having great difficulties with their children or partners and brought those problems to the nursing home to discuss with each other. Overall, the boundaries between home and work issues were very permeable. The volunteers found it acceptable and desirable to talk to one another about what was happening at home. The spillover from family to work served as connecting threads for working together and establishing trust.

Esther's 16-year-old son had been arrested and incarcerated during that winter. She complained of stress and the inability to concentrate on the job: *"I'm lightheaded, I can't sleep, I stay up and cry all night, and I don't want to come here."* She frequently experienced anxiety and other symptoms that caused her to leave the worksite early. Having been recently reunited with her children, she was learning how to recognize asthmatic symptoms and hyperactive symptoms in her sons, but she was so overwhelmed at work worrying about them. She told me one afternoon, *"I don't know what to do. I need advice."*

Dolores's oldest son also was incarcerated. The mother of his son was JoAnn, a peer with whom Dolores worked, and this family complication within the work relationship caused Dolores great stress. It was hard to separate work issues from the powerful feelings between JoAnn and Dolores that revolved around the issues of their children.

Connie and Betty brought their family problems directly into the setting by bringing their children to the site. On several of my visits to the nursing home, Connie had her young son challenged with Erbs Palsy along side her as she worked. The volunteers would discuss how to help him become more independent in dressing and how to get the services needed for his therapy. Connie had a legal case to try to be compensated for her son's disability, and the volunteers would joke that Connie would be "a rich woman." But in the interim, they tried to help her find solutions to her problems while they fed the residents.

Betty often brought her girls to the site after their medical appointments, because if she had brought them back to school, she would have had to miss work. On Friday afternoons, when sitting with their residents who were watching a movie, the volunteers would talk with Betty about her most recent problems with her daughters. Controlling television programming and after-school recreation were frequent topics.

Florence and Agnes kept their private lives out of the work setting more than the other participants did. When they experienced problems at home, they managed to get permission to leave the site and take care of their problems at home. They did not use the volunteer group to help with their home issues.

STAGE 5: STRUGGLING WITH THE SYSTEM.

Struggling with the system involved rectifying the system's mistakes relating to the welfare benefits of baby-sitting money, rent money, food stamps, or Medicaid. The slightest mistake or inconsistency could result in a family's being off balance. At some point in the program, frequently during moving from one program to another, the volunteers had to cope with a serious system error. Florence had been taken off the system when her time was over at the nursing home, but several months later she was still at home waiting for reassignment.

Esther had lost her food stamp benefit once she reunited with her four children; she was without this benefit for four months and had to fight to get it back. She also had to fight for Medicaid benefits for her young son, who needed treatment for asthma and Attention Deficit Hyperactive Disorder (ADHD). Connie was frequently in trouble because the system had not paid her rent or sent food stamps. During these times, she relied on the help of others.

Both Agnes and Dolores had the least problems with the system. Although Agnes found that the system's inconsistent method for paying her threw her off balance, she had a recommendation for what would improve the system: Instead of a benefit, give the volunteers a real job and pay them weekly so that they can manage their expenses. Dolores had a home business and seemed the least stressed by the inconsistencies of the system.

STAGE 6: CONTEMPLATING CHANGES FOR THE BETTER

Contemplating changes refers to the process of reflection that integrated the disappointments in the past and present with the hopes for the future. Holding onto hope and also faith in a higher power enabled the volunteers to use examining their pasts as a tool to improve their children's lives. Based on their past experiences, they made promises to themselves about their present and future maternal responsibility and work.

Betty looked back on her childhood with both tears and laughter. Recognition that her life's early problems were being repeated in her present led her to consider what would happen to her young daughters if they remained in an unsafe home environment. By the end of this study, Betty was contemplating sending her children to their father's homeland. "*I want to save them.*" Knowing her dedication to her children and how much of a loss it would be not to have them nearby indicated just how much she had changed. She was starting to accept the dangerous reality of her situation and was considering ways to remove herself from the environment. In some ways, however, Betty contemplated not changing. Rather than go into a training program or take a private duty job, she preferred to stick to the program rather than risk losing her benefit.

Esther began to consider the possibility of taking her children to visit the home of her maternal family in the South. She wanted her children to experience a sense of roots, a connection she herself was missing.

Dolores wanted to become literate. Family literacy became a goal at home. Structuring study time for the children, learning from them, watching educational programs, going to the library to look at books were activities that helped Dolores move toward literacy. Realizing that her benefit would be finished within a year, she saw herself volunteering because she enjoyed helping people and working on the home business with her husband. Of all the participants, Dolores was the least anxious about the benefit ending.

Agnes contemplated leaving the nursing home. Working with the residents, coupled with caring for her mother, became too depressing for her to tolerate. She considered changing directions in her career path and planned to try a program in which she would learn nontraditional skills, such as construction, painting, or engineering.

Connie was disappointed in the lack of progress in finding a job, and she felt she had wasted a year at the nursing home. She decided that she needed to be more focused, and when she returned to the nursing home again, she was determined to ask for what she wanted, a more structured experience in nursing. Having been taken off the roster, Florence had been waiting for reassignment. Eventually, she was reassigned to a sanitation site, but rather than accept an assignment she did not want, she appealed. She decided to stand up for her principle of choice. She believed that the problem with the program was that people needed to be given choices in what they were interested in. She was setting an example for others.

REFLECTIONS ON STRUGGLES/CRISES IN DYNAMIC PROCESSES

In this chapter, I described six thematic lived aspects of forced transition. The aspects are not linear, but they are dynamic processes through which the volunteers moved during their experiences at the work site, and their responses to each lived aspect were always interwoven with their family life. In addition, I will also describe the counterparts embedded within each stage in order to provide a more holistic description of the participant's experience.

The counterpart of compliance is resistance. Sometimes the volunteers described the nature of their resistance at the beginning of the program, such as not wanting to attend or having a negative attitude toward the program. It is important for administrators of workfare programs to understand that whereas some volunteers may be able to comply, others will resist and may be in need of particular interventions to help them adjust to the program.

The counterpart to engagement in activities is withdrawal. Esther demonstrated this underside of engagement in activities. She was bored and did not enjoy working with the ill residents. She avoided resident contact and would sometimes move around without a particular task objective. One possible cause of her reported boredom was related to not having enough training or supervision to provide purposeful activities for the residents. Low literacy levels also made it difficult to participate in leading activities that required reading instructions. Rather than ask for help, some volunteers would withdraw by sitting away from the residents or responding like Esther.

The counterpart to conflict with authority is conflict resolution. The volunteers and the staff needed learning techniques to constructively negotiate conflict. Training in conflict resolution would have helped Connie and Dolores in their dilemma with Camilla (Ury, 1991, Fisher & Ury, 1981). Although Connie used whatever resources she had to cope with her negative feelings toward Camilla, she was unable to have her needs met for training. Perhaps if Dolores had had some training in conflict resolution, she would have been able to stay at the nursing home rather than leave out of fear that her rage at Camilla would lead her back to prison.

The counterpart to family-work spillover is work-family spillover or bringing home the troubles from work into the home. Problems with feeling demoralized and unrecognized were connected with the volunteers reporting feelings of depression in their work. Already tired from the labor-intensive work, negative feelings spilled over from work to home.

The counterpart to struggling with the system is getting through the system. System errors complicated the work situation, causing much frustration in the home life of Florence, Esther and Connie when they were taken off the program. Learning to negotiate with welfare workers and workfare trainers was necessary to obtaining benefits such as food stamps, Medicaid, and appropriate workfare placements. Getting through the system required perseverance, diplomacy, and having a support network until things were back in place.

The counterpart to contemplating change is evaluation and goal-setting. Given the diverse experiences of each participant in the program, contemplating change occurred after understanding that either they would not get a job in the nursing home or that one's domestic life situation that was having a negative impact on the workfare experience was not changing for the better. There is an opportunity within the workfare set-ting for helping volunteers voice any changes they are contemplating and turning them into purposeful action through evaluating needs and abilities and then helping volunteers set goals for present and future achievement. Betty would have been helped enormously if she could have talked about the dangerous situation in her home, her need for help with her daughters, her wish to become more educated, and her desire to eventually open up a program for women like herself. Had she gone through a process of evaluation of skills and goal-setting, perhaps she would have contemplated other scenarios than having to beg and live in the streets when her time was up.

doi:10.1300/J004v23n03_10

Chapter 11

Holding It All Together

SUMMARY. In this chapter, I answer the research questions and discuss the findings of the qualitative study. doi:10.1300/J004v23n03_11 *[Article copies available for a fee from The Haworth Document Delivery Service: 1-800-HAWORTH. E-mail address: <docdelivery@haworthpress.com> Website: <http://www.HaworthPress.com> © 2007 by The Haworth Press, Inc. All rights reserved.]*

KEYWORDS. Program preparation, resource factors, support, coping, distress, multiple barriers

INTRODUCTION

In this chapter, I answer the research questions noted at the end of Chapter 1 with the data that emerged from the data analysis. I discuss the findings in light of both the 1974 to 1997 literature reviewed in Chapter 2, as well as the latest information on TANF outcomes also addressed in Chapter 2.

[Haworth co-indexing entry note]: "Holding It All Together." Greer, Ellen. Co-published simultaneously in *Occupational Therapy in Mental Health* (The Haworth Press, Inc.) Vol. 23. No. 3/4, 2007, pp. 153-165; and: *Women's Immersion in a Workfare Program: Emerging Challenges for Occupational Therapists* (Ellen Greer) The Haworth Press. 2007, pp. 153-165. Single or multiple copies of this article are available for a fee from The Haworth Document Delivery Service [1-800-HAWORTH, 9:00 a.m. - 5:00 p.m. (EST). E-mail address: docdelivery@haworthpress.com].

RESEARCH QUESTION 1

How do these women receiving TANF experience the mandatory work program as preparation for transition into the workforce?

Perlmutter (1997) points out that prior to the Personal Responsibility Work Reconciliation Act (PRWRA) in 1996, the objective of welfare training programs was to train welfare recipients for employment. However, the objective of the PRWRA initiative regarding work and work-related programs is quick job preparation and placement strategy.

This study suggests that the mandated work program was not geared toward quick job preparation and placement. TANF participants could repeat the program over many cycles without ever transitioning into a job. While the program offered a job search module and classes on resume writing skills, many participants lacked the literacy level required to accomplish such tasks.

From another perspective, research on program evaluation (Gueron & Pauley, 1991) found that those individuals moderately disadvantaged made the largest earning gains when entering the work force. This study found that the participants in the mandated work program at the nursing home were severely disadvantaged by multiple barriers (e.g., literacy, history of abuse, food insecurity, and housing insecurity) and did not make the transition to sustained employment. Florence reported that she had a two-week job as a health care aide while waiting to be reassigned to the mandated program. Esther had a seasonal job collecting tickets at an amusement park and was able to have Betty hired for three weeks in the summer. Dolores worked as a baby-sitter and had a small business with her husband. The intermittent work found by these four participants was not the result of the mandated work program.

Gueron and Pauley (1991) also found that mothers with young children had great difficulty making the transition to work and maintaining sustained employment. In most cases, the participants in this study had young and teenage children with multiple needs for educational, psychosocial, and health attention, and I found that mothers with teenage children were more stressed than were mothers with younger children. Having teenagers who were not going to school or who were experiencing mental health and physical health crisis created enormous conflicts for those mothers who had to attend the mandated program.

In most cases, participants' relatives helped with the younger children, providing a more secure child-care arrangement. Connie's young child was cared for by her mother-in-law. Florence's children were picked up from the bus by their aunt who lived with them. Dolores's young son was supervised by his father, who worked at home. Esther's sister followed up on the supervision of her younger sons.

Wittman, Staham and Rhoades (1997) suggest that the effectiveness of mandated work programs needs further investigation to meet the needs of poor families with young children. This study suggests that poor mothers with teenagers need professional support in meeting the parenting demands of their children, as well as strategies to manage their individual distress levels in daily life at home and in the mandated work program.

The Association of Maternal Child Health Programs (2002) propose that state welfare programs take a role in developing programs to reduce adolescent risk factors, as well as protect women and families.

Diverse Participant Perspectives

The participants had diverse opinions as to whether the mandated program prepared them for the workforce. Table 2 depicts their points of view and the obstacles that they viewed to be in their way.

Esther was the only participant who believed she was not prepared for the workforce. The other participants felt the mandated program provided them with opportunities to learn new skills, and for several volunteers with previous experience in caring for the elderly, this was just additional practice in an area in which they already felt comfortable.

However, these participants still identified the following obstacles to obtaining a job: lack of education, history of incarceration, lack of specialized training, lack of money for certification tests. Four participants

TABLE 2. Participants' Perspectives on Program Preparation and Obstacles

Participant	Prepared	Obstacle
Esther	No	Lack of literacy skills; stigma of drug, prison, and welfare
Florence	Yes	Lack of Funds for nurse's assistant certification exam; welfare stigma
Dolores	Yes	Lack of literacy skills; stigma of drug, prison, and welfare
Betty	Yes	Lack of literacy skills; stigma of arrest, and welfare
Agnes	Yes	Lack of training that will lead to a job; welfare stigma
Connie	Yes	Lack of literacy skills; stigma of drug, prison, and welfare

found education to be the primary barrier, believing that two days of school per week was not adequate preparation to meet the literacy requirements demanded in a work setting. Dolores and Connie were coping with English as a second language. Although Agnes and Florence had the credentials to begin college, they could not because of the threat of losing the TANF benefit.

Three of those four participants also faced obstacles due to a history of drugs and incarceration. They had to deal with fingerprint identification when applying for certain jobs, particularly in the area of child-care, and they tended to avoid any job interview that would require a formal background check. Dolores coped by creating her own micro enterprise, Esther found itinerant seasonal work and Connie hoped that one day having a college degree would help her get a good job. Although their histories included difficult circumstances to explain to an employer, the women did not have the needed legal knowledge about their human rights in making this transition from welfare to work. Without legal advice, they were acting on what they feared, while they may have had other options open to them.

Training and certification was an issue for two participants. Both Agnes and Florence had their GED and were concerned about obtaining the training and certification necessary to get a job with a livable wage. The other four participants were primarily concerned with education.

All of the participants were affected by welfare stigma. Their status as TANF recipients caused stress in the workplace, as they experienced being treated with disrespect or lack of recognition. The dread of feeling the shame of their welfare status inhibited perusing job interviews. As Betty remarked, *"How am I going to explain what I have been doing? I don't want to tell them I'm on welfare–you understand?"*

RESEARCH QUESTION 2

How do women fit this mandatory program into daily life?

Fitting the mandated program into daily life required complex negotiation in performing multiple tasks that are part of motherwork–running a household, caring for other kin, and finding leisure time for play and relaxation. Tasks suffering the most were the levels of attention that needed to be directed to the care and supervision of their children. Holding things together to maintain all the requirements to receive the TANF benefit led to paying less attention to child supervision, such as homework, because of fatigue or because it was important to spend time on keeping the house in good shape to protect against sanctions by a BCW worker.

Participants arrived at the worksite at 9:00 am and left at 4:30 pm. All the women had to ready their children in the morning before coming to the worksite, and would return home at approximately 5:30 pm to join their families. Evenings were spent preparing dinner, cleaning the house, and readying the children for bed. All of the participants described themselves as being too tired in the evening to help the children with their homework. Given that five days a week the women were busy almost 10 hours a day traveling to the nursing home, working the entire day, and traveling home, they were left with approximately 5 to 6 hours to spend with their families before bedtime. The weekends became a time for fitting in many activities–maintenance of clothing, child-care, self-care, supervision of children's homework, doing their own homework, playing with their children, leisure activities, other paid work, looking for shelter, talking on the phone, and prayer. A more detailed discussion of how they spent their time is presented below.

Resource Factors

Time, support, and coping strategies helped participants meet their basic needs for physical survival and emotional safety and thus to comply with the mandated work program.

Time

Time was a major factor in incorporating the mandated work program into daily life. Activities took place on the weekends, before work, lunchtime, after work, and late evenings.

All the participants except Ann set aside supermarket excursions for the weekends. Betty had a Dollar Van in her neighborhood that took her to the supermarket in the early evening after work. Other activities that participants left for the weekends included housecleaning, playing with children, leisure activities, other paid work, child-care grooming (i.e., hair washing and braiding), and maintenance of clothing (i.e., washing, ironing, and sewing).

In the mornings before work, all of the participants had to ready their children for school. Only Florence mentioned cooking breakfast for her children each morning. Betty discussed her problems with her young teenage daughter not wanting to leave for school and often having to leave her home alone in order to arrive at work on time.

Participants used lunchtime to meet their own needs. They frequently ate a meal either brought from home or purchased from the nursing home or an outside deli or fast-food restaurant. Sometimes they needed to find a check-cashing establishment to cash their TANF benefit. Purchasing clothing or toys from vendors inside and outside of the nursing home was part of the lunch hour ritual, and eventually buying jewelry from a vendor who began visiting the nursing home became a high point of the day. Because the participants could pay for the jewelry in installments, it became an accessible activity that brought about friendly social interactions with the nursing home staff, who were doing the same thing.

Lunchtime was also a break in the day when a participant could sign out should she need to take care of personal business related to their child's schooling or related to welfare (e.g., going to the welfare office for an interview or complain about missing benefits). If the participant did not feel well and could not function in the setting any longer that day, lunchtime was the hour to leave after obtaining Dorothea's permission.

The major activities conducted after work included cooking dinner, engaging in self-care routines to relax, monitoring children's homework, and completing one's own homework if fatigue had not taken over. Straightening up the home was also part of everyone's daily activities; however, Betty reported that every day was like "*spring cleaning,*" meaning she washed the walls and floors down every day. To relax, she would "*lay back*" with her daughter and later watch the 11:00 o'clock news to find out the next day's weather.

Connie went home after work before she picked up her toddler son. Once home, she took a bath to unwind, would proceed to make dinner for her two older sons, and then go to pick up the youngest. Once she returned home again, she prepared the toddler for bed and later focused on helping her school-age sons complete their homework.

Caring for relatives also was provided after work. Agnes described coming to the nursing home, then leaving at the end of the day to run and take care of her mother, and then finally to go home to take care of her family.

Talking on the phone to discuss the day's problems with friends and family or to make plans for the week with peers from the nursing home was part of an evening's range of activities. Betty, Esther, Connie, and Dolores spoke on the phone to each other frequently during weekday evenings. The hours after work and the weekends were most significant in meeting personal needs for self and the family.

Support

Support consisted of social/emotional, physical, educational, and material resources. Social/emotional support was found within the nuclear family unit and sometimes extended to grandmothers. Most participants explained that when they needed support, they could only count on their immediate family. Florence and Connie received social/emotional support from their mothers, and Esther counted on her older sister. Other study participants relied on their bonds with their children.

Unlike Stack's study (1974), which suggested that poor families established flexible networks with kin and unrelated kin in fostering reciprocity, the participants in this study had very limited networks in care giving for the children and limited shared resources with kin and unrelated kin (friends). Belle (1994) found that poor women who had previously been middle class had greater resources from their middle-class families, while poor women who had grown up in poverty had minimal resources and supports from their families and often were the ones to provide support when necessary. In contrast to Belle's research, this study found that TANF participants experienced reciprocity in social/emotional supports between themselves and their families. Material resources were limited, and the participants could not count on their kin for material support.

Social-Emotional Support

In times when professional help was clearly needed, participants turned to family, friends, or peers at work to avoid exposing their problems to authorities who could punish them by taking away their children. In discussing Betty's dilemma about leaving her daughter who had had hip surgery, Dolores tried to persuade Ann to seek help from BCW. Although she was in desperate need of help, Betty ignored that advice because she knew that she would jeopardize her family.

Physical Support

Family members provided physical assistance in activities. Florence's oldest daughter was learning how to cook and would occasionally assist her mother in meal preparation. Betty's older children cleaned the apartment after she had complained that they were not helping, but instead of this being a relief, she was dissatisfied with their housecleaning: "*I have to go and clean up everything they cleaned.*" Dolores's husband helped with the baby-sitting and supervision of the children. Esther and Agnes had older children who were capable of helping around the house. Except for Dolores's husband and Florence's aunt, the participants lacked having another adult in the home environment with them to share the burden of multiple responsibilities. This translated into their coming home from work at the nursing home extremely fatigued to attend to their families.

Educational Support

Educational support came from the programs in which participants were preparing for the GED. They were able to apply the literacy skills they were refining to the family unit, either by helping their children with homework whenever possible or doing their own homework. With increased knowledge and skills, their scope of activities and their plans for the future opened up. Dolores focused on family literacy, thus expanding cultural activities in the home. Florence learned advanced nursing skills that would prepare her for an eventual career in nursing. Esther and Betty, while struggling with basic literacy skills, learned to read and found themselves becoming more comfortable talking to their children about their homework. Connie used her enhanced literacy skills from the program to help her two sons learn to cope with English as a second language. Agnes was determined to set an example for her daughters by not only earning her GED, but by having her knowledge base be even larger than theirs.

For Agnes, Connie, Betty, Esther and Dolores, having an understanding teacher who encouraged them and gave them opportunities to learn was a significant and empowering educational support. In this respect, the mandated program was pivotal in their increased literacy.

Material Support

The major source of material support (money) came from the TANF benefit. Receiving the baby-sitting income provided them with enough money to either pay a childcare worker to stay with the children at home or to pay for a day-care program. In those cases where participants decided to have older children care for the younger children, the income was used for basic necessities, such as clothing and shoes. Having some kind of child-care arrangement in place cost money, even if the caretaker was a family member other than the older children. With appropriate child-care arrangements, the participants were able to come to work with minimal worry. Except for Betty who faced a dilemma in child-care (see

Chapter 9), the benefit supported satisfactory child-care arrangements for the participants.

Coping

Kelly and Voyandorf (1985) looked at two types of role strain that occur from working mothers performing multiple roles: overload and interference. Overload is more prescribed activities than an individual can handle; interference is conflict between rote expectation and having to do two things simultaneously. These two concepts are relevant in the discussion of how this study's participants fit the workfare program into their lives.

The breakdown in handling the activities in one's life revolved around the participants' being too tired from the workday to help their children with homework in the evenings. Increased working hours left less time at home to attend to family needs, as well as to meet their own responsibilities as GED students with homework assignments.

Conflict over wanting to be in two places at one time was frequently related to the well-being of their children. Florence described being conflicted when her child was sick. She could stay home and not be sanctioned if she took her daughter to the doctor and got a doctor's note as documentation; however, she realized that sometimes her child did not need immediate medical attention and perhaps needed to just rest out a cold. In those situations, Florence felt she should stay home, but she would still come to work.

Betty faced the conflict of interference every day when she left her teenage daughter at home who refused to go to school. She wanted to be home and available to help her, but she also wanted to fulfill her workfare obligation. Unfortunately, she was in a dilemma. If she could not get her child to school, she was in danger of losing her daughters, and if she stayed home to deal with the problem, she would lose her benefit.

I believe that because the participants had to live with daily threats of losing their children if they did not comply with TANF regulations, then the concept of role-strain does not encompass their actual experience. I suggest the construct be expanded to *role-distress,* which incorporates the added component of threat in performing both roles of mother and workfare participant.

In facing the multiple demands in their roles as mothers, daughters, partners, workfare workers, and students, the participants were challenged by high levels of stress. When Esther's oldest son was going before a judge for adjudication, she described the pain of the experience in watching her son moving towards incarceration. She explained how she stayed up nights crying, unable to sleep, and had an extremely difficult time coming to the nursing home in the morning. Yet, she fit the program into her life, even when her home life was threatened. She coped by gathering the support from her workfare peers, Betty, Connie, and Dolores, who understood her predicament, for each had had experiences of personal and family incarceration.

Agnes had multiple care giving demands. She was a one-to-one companion to Alice in the nursing home, and after work she would visit her mother who lived with the residuals of a stroke. Feeling exceedingly burdened and saddened from caring for elderly people who were going to die, Agnes coped by changing her career direction and moved into a program unrelated to caregiving. She had reached a point where she could no longer emotionally fit the program into her life, and she had chosen to maintain her benefit by transferring into another program.

Dolores had many pressures in the workplace. She had an in-law relationship with Dorothea, she questioned Camilla's authority, and she had been accused of stealing her own records. From experience, she knew that if she expressed her anger, she could end up in prison. She could no longer fit the program into her life, and she left. Because she wanted to maintain the TANF benefit, she asked for another placement. Dolores coped by knowing her own behavior and made a choice to be placed into a more neutral environment.

Coping with difficult life situations created opportunities for the participants to respond with resilience. A resilient response did not necessarily mean that the participant would continue to fit the program into her daily life if the situation was negative for her. In some cases, as in that of Agnes and Dolores, the participant had to choose to leave the program and begin again somewhere else. The nature of these coping strategies revolved around relational interactions of connection (bonding with others) disconnection (isolating from others), transcendence (relation with a higher power through prayer), and assertive problem solving.

Both Florence and Connie had been taken out of the program because of system errors. They handled the situation by asking the program supervisor for the workfare assignments they wanted. Florence found necessary part-time employment and enhanced her home life and mothering role. Both women reflected on what they needed to do to progress.

Most of all, Betty demonstrated a commitment to her workfare assignment and survival for herself and her children. She gained strength from prayer, and her practical knowledge taught her how to get what she needed from the work setting. Her desire to survive shaped how she was able to fit in the workfare program every day, even when her family was in turmoil. As she said about her workfare assignment, *"It is my bread and water."*

Rank (1994) found that individuals who received welfare benefits had several coping strategies that helped them deal with the barriers they faced–psychological stigma, problems within and outside the family, and structural class differences. He identified faith, resilience, and determination as the dominant coping strategies. Each of these three coping strategies was described by the participants in the context of everyday life. Responding with resilience and staying committed to the program with determined purpose was found in the stories of Ann, Florence, Dolores, Connie, Agnes. and Esther, while only Betty, Florence, and Connie spoke about practicing faith in God. It was clear, however, that Esther, Dolores, and Agnes had faith and a strong value system to do good for their children and society. However, in contrast to Rank's findings, the participants also coped through relational strategies with their peers in the mandated work setting, helping each other with domestic parenting and work issues.

RESEARCH QUESTION 3

How do these women feel about this transition into the workforce?

The way that Connie answered this question represented the core attitude of the participants: *"We are willing and wanting but not getting a chance."* Underlying Connie's statement was her belief that the participants were motivated and desired to make the transition, but they could not do it on their own. In fact, the system was not giving them the appropriate chance for success.

Working through initial resistances in making the transition to workfare and growing in the direction of cooperation gave the participants confidence that they could master difficult situations and indeed succeed in the work environment. Yet feelings of frustration and demoralization conflicted with those of satisfaction and self-esteem, creating overall ambivalence. Fear and uncertainty about the future (being taken out of the system without a job) was always an undermining force that enhanced the general ambivalence.

Frustration emerged whenever the participants were led to believe their actions would lead to work but then were ultimately let down, either by false promises, errors in the system, or the lack of necessary resources to finish a training program. Demoralization was a response to feeling continually unrecognized, unappreciated, and disrespected by the nursing home staff.

The participants were determined to make the best of the opportunity and learn as much as they could in their workfare assignment at the nursing home. In their interactions with the residents, they discovered their unique capabilities in providing care giving activities and winning the trust of the residents. This led to feelings of satisfactory performance. Over time, the participants experienced self-esteem as they became more confident and independent in carrying out activities with the residents. This was evident in the change in their appearance, from dressing casually in jeans to more professional attire.

In presenting their points of view, it was clear that the participants valued their past histories and successes in surviving. Using their knowledge from past experience on how to survive helped them connect with each other and the residents for whom they cared through compassion for the vulnerability of others. They highly valued this quality they had developed. Toward the end of the study, Betty, Esther, and Connie had transformed themselves from laid-back volunteers to volunteers with a voice regarding the care of the residents. Not only did they recognize what was wrong, but they suggested how to improve care. They were no longer afraid or intimidated by what the staff thought of them.

The forced transition from welfare status to workfare brought fear and uncertainty regarding real problems in the present and anticipated problems in the future. Fears expressed by the participants centered around loss of food and shelter, loss of children to BCW, and loss of emotional well-being because of financial difficulties.

Uncertainty pervaded everyday life. A free-floating anxiety of an unknown threat permeated the participants' lives. They were never sure where they were going next. The anxiety underneath the uncertainty was evident in Esther's question, *"What will happen to us?"* In the most positive and determined narrative, Agnes stated she was going to get a job, yet she revealed her fear of being homeless if she did not get a job. Florence, who had advanced the farthest in her training, fought against the fear of being homeless if things did not work out. Esther could not imagine how she would be able to find a paid job to provide for her family without an adequate education. She could not believe that "they" (the system) would not help her.

The underlying fear of being abandoned by the system and potentially losing their families to foster care was connected to each participant's past experiences of being abandoned by their mothers and fathers in varying circumstances. When they were children, there had been grandparents or institutions to take over the parental functions. Now, in this transition, the participants were preparing to lose the symbolic caretaker ("welfare"), and although they wanted to make it on their own and be self-sufficient, they may not have been ready because of unresolved multiple barriers.

The following five multiple barriers were associated with raising frustration and demoralization, as well as the anxiety from fear and uncertainty. Although the participants also experienced satisfaction and self-esteem in their transitional process of working with the nursing home residents and the slow gain of literacy skills, those feelings were not powerful enough to reduce their levels of distress in face of adversity.

- Serious psychosocial and medical problems with children and adolescents in the family
- Lack of adequate preparation in developing literacy skills in reading and writing
- Stigma from history of welfare, incarceration and drug abuse
- No child-care provisions for teenagers
- Threat of food and housing insecurity

The conflict between being job ready (expressed by the attitude, "We are willing and wanting but not getting the chance") and the fear of being rejected by the outside world (expressed by disappointment in a system that is not helping them) is strengthened by the multiple barriers interwoven in everyday life. Such opposing tensions in the forced transition from welfare to workfare created an overall sense of ambivalence in the participants, expressed as either wanting to move ahead or to just run away. Overall, the participants tolerated these difficult feelings about the transition to work and did what was necessary to maintain their benefit and their families.

doi:10.1300/J004v23n03_11

Chapter 12

What I Have Learned:
Conclusions

SUMMARY. In this chapter I revisit the goals of TANF in light of the findings of this research study and present recommendations for policy change. doi:10.1300/J004v23n03_12 *[Article copies available for a fee from The Haworth Document Delivery Service: 1-800-HAWORTH. E-mail address: <docdelivery@haworthpress.com> Website: <http://www.HaworthPress.com> © 2007 by The Haworth Press, Inc. All rights reserved.]*

KEYWORDS. TANF, workfare policy, adolescent care-care provisions, educational options for mothers, financial and work provisions, occupational therapy

Seeking to establish a new basis of security and prosperity . . . regardless of station or race or creed, FDR called for "a second Bill of Rights" that would guarantee:

[Haworth co-indexing entry note]: "What I Have Learned: Conclusions." Greer, Ellen. Co-published simultaneously in *Occupational Therapy in Mental Health* (The Haworth Press, Inc.) Vol. 23, No. 3/4, 2007, pp. 167-173; and: *Women's Immersion in a Workfare Program: Emerging Challenges for Occupational Therapists* (Ellen Greer) The Haworth Press, 2007, pp. 167-173. Single or multiple copies of this article are available for a fee from The Haworth Document Delivery Service [1-800-HAWORTH, 9:00 a.m. - 5:00 p.m. (EST). E-mail address: docdelivery@haworthpress.com].

The right to a useful and remunerative job; The right to earn enough to provide adequate food and clothing and recreation; The right . . . to a decent home; The right to adequate medical care and the opportunity to achieve and enjoy good health; The right to adequate protection from the economic fears of old age and sickness and accident and unemployment and . . . The right to a good education.

Social policy in the United States has never approached this vision. As a nation, we remain at a great distance from the system of economic justice advocated by President Roosevelt 50 years ago. Yet the rights of the poor have increased during the intervening years, and largely because of the struggles of poor people themselves.

Hershkoff & Loffredeo (1997, p. xv)

INTRODUCTION

The goals of TANF as authorized by the Personal Responsibility and Work Opportunity Reconciliation Act of 1996 as defined by Congress are (1) to provide temporary assistance to needy families with children, subject to tough work requirements and time-limited eligibility; (2) to discourage poor women from having children out of wedlock and to encourage the formation of marital families; and (3) to ensure that needy adults work so that their families can become self-sufficient (Hershkoff & Loffredeo, 1997). But how well did these goals measure up according to the experiences of the six female participants in this study?

Workfare as an intervention provided a method and structure to implement the first goal. Indeed, the work requirements were tough and time-limited. However, there was no mechanism within the program to process the problems and difficulties that the participants encountered.

As for the second goal, no participants became pregnant or married during the year that I talked with them. Florence and Agnes could no longer bear children. Betty, Esther, Connie, and Dolores had completed their families and never discussed the possibility of having another child. They were focused on meeting the current needs of their children and were often burdened by the medical and psychosocial problems that required their attention.

Dolores was the only participant who had a partner living with her. Betty's husband, who had been deported to the Caribbean after nine years of incarceration, lived very poorly in his country. Betty often struggled with whether she should send her children to live with him. When circumstances in her family life felt hopeless and as the time limits approached signaling the end of her TANF benefit, Betty spoke about living with her husband in a hut, where she would sleep on the earthen floor.

The father of Florence's children needed a visa and a green card to enter the country. Florence was not ready to sponsor him and was resolved to raise her children on her own. She believed that a woman should be able to make it on her own because a man could leave her–or die–at any time. Esther's partner, the father of her children, was in and out of her life. Early in their relationship, they had abused drugs together. Having made a complete recovery, Esther was distressed that he continued to use drugs. Although she depended on him for material resources, she felt a strong need to disconnect from the relationship not only because of his drug abuse, but also because of his likely betrayal with another woman.

Connie's husband was serving time in prison on the East Coast. Her young boys missed their father, but Connie found it increasingly difficult to visit him on the weekends with the children because of the drain on time and emotions.

Agnes had separated from her husband two years earlier at the time she had become a TANF recipient. The father of her daughters, he maintained contact with them and provided material support. At the time of the interviews, Agnes was having a relationship with a new man whom she liked and trusted. She worked exceedingly hard to help her daughters accept her right to have a boyfriend.

It appears that TANF encouraged some of these participants to remain in relationships with men who provided some financial support or protection but these were not satisfying relationships. Perhaps if Betty, Connie, Esther, and Florence actually transitioned into sustained employment in which they earned a living wage, they would consider other marriage options or alternative family styles, such as getting divorced or living with a community of friends who supported one another and cared for each other's children.

The third goal of TANF–to ensure that needy adults work and enable their families to be self-sufficient–was not met. The workfare participants were repeatedly cycling through the program, with no bridge leading to sustained employment. Instead of strengthening the families, the constant system errors, inadequate amount of food stamps, and insecure housing situations seemed to make the families who had already been needy because of multiple barriers all the more vulnerable.

REFLECTIONS ON PARTICIPANTS' STATE OF DISTRESS

What I find most interesting about my findings is just how distant TANF is from fulfilling President Franklin D. Roosevelt's proposed second bill of rights. Society must move closer to meeting the basic human rights of those living in poverty–food and housing security, a job with a livable wage, and freedom from the fear of economic insecurity. The findings of my study suggest that the participants in the mandated work program felt prepared to make the transition to work, but they also felt held back by multiple barriers not addressed in the program. Given the pervasive threat and uncertainty about their future, along with insecurity about food and housing and the overarching fear of losing their children, the participants appear to be in a state of distress, as defined by the American Psychological Association (1998). Compounding their domestic role-distress was the threatening feelings of marginalization, for in the work setting, the participants were being treated as an underclass labor pool.

Individuals in distress are at risk for physical and emotional illness, thus placing their children at risk, as well. Without adequate supports, it is unlikely that the intergenerational cycle will be broken for workfare participants. At the start of my research, the women told me that they continued going around in a circle and wanted to see some type of change. I now understand the intensity of their frustration of wanting to improve their life, but no matter what they did, no matter how much they cooperated with the system, they could not make any significant changes; in fact, their life could become worse. Why is society asking poor mothers to do the impossible without the necessary external supports, but then blaming them for not becoming self-sufficient? From this study, I learned that the problem is not a lack of desire on the participants' part, but rather a lack of different programs for women with diverse and special needs.

The women in this study were mothers living in poverty. Among the 6 women were 20 children, of which over 80% were failing in school. Our question should really be how welfare reform can help mothers do their first and primary job, which is raising children to be good citizens. Welfare reform should not only enable poor women with multiple barriers to be successful in their transition to work, but it should also support them in their role as mothers.

Adversity can sometimes be a good thing. It can bring out one's creativity in coping with difficult life situations; it can strengthen ego and family resilience. Yet sometimes adversity can tip an individual over into illness, depression, or crime.

My Personal Experience with Adversity

When I first started this study, I viewed myself as a middle-class white women of privilege; by the time I ended this study, my view changed to being a woman who, because she had struggled with adversity, felt more connected to the universal struggle that women face as mothers and as individuals in sickness and health. I now realize that viewing myself as different had been a way to keep myself separate and distanced from my participants.

Like the participants, I, too, had a teenage child who was struggling to find his path. Often my feelings of frustration and despair resonated with those of the participants, but I did not share with them the details of the difficulties I was experiencing in my own motherwork. At times, I felt like a sister to the participants, and I yearned for the closeness and ease that they had found with one another.

Later, after the interviews had been conducted, I was diagnosed with breast cancer. Now it was my turn to taste the uncertainty and fear of not knowing one's future. Going within to find my deepest well of courage and strength was not enough. I needed supports of all kinds to make it through–medical, emotional, and spiritual.

What I have come to understand is that success requires interdependence between the individual who needs help and the individual who is giving the help as they work together. It is a delicate balance, a profound interaction, and an opportunity to promote growth. In order for this interdependence to occur, the policy lens that influences the lives of TANF families has to be changed.

RECOMMENDATIONS FOR WORKFARE POLICY CHANGES

The findings of this study lead me to suggest the following policy changes.

ADOLESCENT CHILD-CARE PROVISIONS

1. Provide an educational curriculum for parents that includes both adolescent development classes that focus on didactic and experiential instruction in the human development of adolescents and also coping strategies to ensure constructive support of their adolescents.
2. Develop community programs and outreach for adolescents in underserved neighborhoods.

3. Provide an economic benefit to pay for child-care or community afterschool educational, health-related, and leisure activities.
4. Provide a mechanism, through interagency collaboration, for an ongoing dialogue between child-care agencies, the police department, and parents of adolescents to foster a working partnership in the interest of the adolescent.

EXPANSION OF EDUCATIONAL OPTIONS FOR MOTHERS

1. Screen for cognitive, emotional, and physical disabilities and refer for an appropriate therapeutic evaluation and treatment plan.
2. Offer full-time educational experiences that lead to mastering basic literacy skills.
3. Assist TANF recipients in making the transition to college or technical training with financial grants to cover basic costs.
4. Train mothers to care for children in their communities, give them a stipend for training, and pay them for the service.

FINANCIAL AND WORK PROVISIONS

1. Use financial incentives that ensure food and housing security as participants go through the transition process.
2. Extend or stop time limits for families who fall into high-risk categories (experiencing psychosocial and medical distress).
3. Reduce the amount of working hours to part-time as an option for mothers who have child-care issues.
4. Consult with TANF mothers on policy issues for improving the transition from welfare to work.
5. Establish an ombudsman role at workfare sites to smooth out glitches between workfare participants and the welfare system.

IMPLICATIONS FOR OCCUPATIONAL THERAPY

Occupational therapists are trained to assist individuals to become independent and self-sufficient. Occupational therapy in the work setting has much to offer TANF recipients in the mandated workfare program, for it can address each individual's unique barriers through evaluation, goal setting, intervention, and re-evaluation.

Using a psycho-educational model, an occupational therapy consultant can address the needs of workfare clients by working closely with an interdisciplinary team of educators, human resource professionals, human rights advocates, legal counsel, social workers, psychologists, psychoanalysts and family therapists, rehabilitation professionals, nutritionists, physicians, nurses and clergy, who together could provide learning modules for the workfare participants either in their workfare setting or the program school setting.

Occupational therapy programs can assist supervisors in workfare settings to ensure the success of their participants. Knowing that participants turn to each other for help is enlightening for choosing an effective intervention. I found that the participants avoided authority and were more comfortable with peer interaction; thus, I recommend that self-help groups addressing topics such as life planning, time management, building support networks, negotiating the system, parent discussion group, and a healthy life-styles/stress-reduction be built into the program, with the consultation of an occupational therapist who facilitates goal-setting and discussion or who can be called upon to address specific individual problems.

FUTURE RESEARCH

This study is just the beginning in understanding the experiences of women in the transition process from welfare to work. It looked directly at the experiences of six women who were recycling through the program without making the transition to sustained employment. Further research needs to examine the experiences of individuals who do make a successful transition to employment so that we can learn what factors made the transition possible. In addition, investigating the experiences of not just adolescents of workfare mothers, but adolescents in general may help determine how to improve the outcome for both mother and child.

I am grateful for the experience of having known the participants in this study. They have taught me so much. I hope that changes in policy and programmatic supports will lift each mother and her family out of poverty and into a safe and secure environment, one that includes rewarding work and enriching relationships–an environment that allows her to be self-sufficient while enjoying the interdependence of connecting with others.

doi:10.1300/J004v23n03_12

Bibliography

Abramovitz, M. (1996). Regulating the lives of women: Social Welfare from colonial times to the present. (Rev. ed.). Boston: South End Press.

Aguilar, M. A., & Williams, L. P. (1993). Factors contributing to the success and achievement of minority women. *Affllia, 8,* 410-424.

American Psychological Association. Public Interest Directorate. (1998). Making 'Welfare to Work' really work. Washington, D. C.: American Psychological Association. Available at http://www.4pa.org/pi/woo/health.html

Aptheker, B. (1989). Tapestries of life: Women's work, women's consciousness, and the meaning of daily experience. Amherst: University of Massachusetts Press.

Association of Maternal Child Health Programs. (2002 March). Principles to protect the health interests of women, children, youth and their families (welfare/tanf reorganization). Fact Sheet. Available at www.amchpl.policy/principlesFS.pdf

Bal, M., Crewe, J., & Spitzer, L. (1999). Acts of memory: Cultural recall in the present. Hanover, NH: Dartmouth College University Press.

Beckman, D. (2002, May 8). The best Mother's Day gift of all. Religion News Service. Washington, DC: Bread for the World. Available at http://www.bread.org/media/articles/2002/religion news service may 8.html

Belle, D. (1994). Attempting to comprehend the lives of low-income women. In C. E. Franz & A. J. Stewart (Eds.). *Women creating lives.* San Franciso: Westview Press.

Berrick, J. D. (1995). Faces of poverty: Portraits of women and children on welfare. New York: Oxford University Press.

Blank, S. W., & Blum, B. B. (1997). A brief history of work expectations for welfare mothers. Welfare to work. *The Future of the Children, 7*(1), 28-38.

Blum, B., & Francis, J. F. (2002). *Welfare research perspectives: Past present and future.* New York: Mailman School of Public Health, Columbia University. Available at www. researchforum.org

Bogdan, R., & Biklin, S. K. (1982). *Qualitative research for education: An introduction to theory and methods.* Boston: Allyn & Bacon.

[Haworth co-indexing entry note]: "Bibliography." Greer, Ellen. Co-published simultaneously in *Occupational Therapy in Mental Health* (The Haworth Press, Inc.) Vol. 23, No. 3/4, 2007, pp. 175-180; and: *Women's Immersion in a Workfare Program: Emerging Challenges for Occupational Therapists* (Ellen Greer) The Haworth Press. 2007, pp. 175-180. Single or multiple copies of this article are available for a fee from The Haworth Document Delivery Service [1-800-HAWORTH, 9:00 a.m. - 5:00 p.m. (EST). E-mail address: docdelivery@haworthpress.com].

Brong, L. (1996). Rebuilding lives: A bridge between welfare and work. *The Humanistic Psychologist, 24,* 383-390.

Bruner, J. (1990). *Acts of meaning.* Cambridge, MA: Harvard University Press.

Campbell, M. L., & Moen, P. (1992). Job-family role strain among employed single mothers of preschoolers. *Family Relations, 41,* 205-211.

Christiansen, K. (1997). With whom so you believe your lot is cast? White feminists and racism. *Signs 22,* 615-648.

Clarke-Kauffman, E., Duncan, G., Gennetian, L., Knox, V., London, A., & Vargas, W. (2002). How welfare and work policies for parents affect adolescents: A synthesis of research. New York: Manpower Demonstration Research Corporation. Available at http://www.mdrc.orp-/publications/69/overview.html

Collins, P. H. (1994). Shifting the center: Race, class and feminist theorizing about motherhood. In D. Bassin, M. Honey, & M. M. Kaplan (Eds.), *Representation of motherhood* (pp. 56-74). New Haven, CT: Yale University Press.

Cortazzi, M. (1993). *Narrative analysis.* London: Falmer Press.

Davis, L. V., & Hagen, J. L. (1996). Stereotypes and stigma: What's changed for welfare mothers. *Affilia, 11,* 319-337.

Delsman, B. (11 August, 1997). A. Bernstein (Interviewer). *Brian Lehrer Show.* New York: WNYC Radio.

Denzin, N. (1989). *Interpretive interactionism: Applied social research method series: Vol. 16.* Thousand Oaks, CA: Sage.

Denzin, N. (1997). *Interpretive ethnography: Ethnographic practices for the 21st century.* Thousand Oaks, CA: Sage.

Edin, K., & Lein, L. (1997). *Making ends meet: How single mothers survive welfare and low-wage work.* New York: Russell Sage Foundation.

Ely, M., Anzul, M., Friedman, T., Garner, D., & Steinmetz, A. (1991). *Doing qualitative research: Circles wrting circles.* London: Falmer Press.

Ely, M., Vinz, R., Downing, M., & Anzul, M. (1997). *On writing qualitative research.* London: Falmer Press.

Enos, S. (2001). *Mothering from inside: Parenting in a women's prison.* Albany: State University of New York Press.

Ensellem, M. (1997). *Welfare reforming the workplace: Protecting the employment rights of welfare recipients, immigrants and displaced workers.* New York: National Employment Law Project.

Fass, S., & Couthen, N. K. (2006). *Who are America's poor children? The official story.* National Center for Children in Poverty (NCCP), Columbia University, Mailman School of Public Health. http://nccp.org/pub_cpt06a.html.

Fisher, R., & Ury, W. (1981). *Getting to yes: Negotiating agreement without giving in.* Boston: Houghton Mifflin.

Future of Children Organization. (2003). *Children and welfare reform: Analysis and recommendations.* Available at http://www.futureofchildren.org

Galtung, J. (1994). *Human rights in another key.* Cambridge, UK: Polity Press.

Gerdes, K. E. (1997). Long-term AFDC mothers and post-traumatic stress syndrome: Is there a connection? *Afflia, 12,* 359-367.

Gerson, K. (1985). *Hard choices: How women decide about work, career, and motherhood.* Los Angeles: University of California Press.

Gilbert, N., Berrick, J. D., & Meyers. M. (1992). *GAIN family life and child care study.* Berkeley: Family Welfare Research Group.

Goldberg, W. A., Greenberger, E. E., Hamill. S., & O'Neill, R. (1992). Role demands in the lives of employed single mothers with preschoolers. *Journal of Family Issues, 13,* 312-333.

Gordimer, N. (1980). *Burger's Daughter.* New York: Penguin Books

Gowdy, E. A., & Pearlmutter, S. (1993). Economic self-sufficiency: It's not just the money. *Affilia, 8,* 368-387.

Grogger, J., & Karoly, L. A. (2005). *Welfare Reform: Effects of a decade of change.* Harvard University Press. A Rand Corporation Study.

Grogger, J., Karoly, L. A., & Klerman, J. A. (2002). *Consequences of welfare reform: A research synthesis.* RAND Child Policy Project, RAND'S Labor and Population Program. (DRU-2676-DHHS). Available at http://www.rand.org/labor/TANF synthesis/

Gueron, J. M., & Pauley, E. (1991). *From welfare to work. A Manpower Demonstration Research Corporation Study.* New York: Russell Sage Foundation.

Herman, J. L. (1992). *Trauma and recovery. The aftermath of violence–from domestic abuse to political terror.* New York: Basic Books.

Hershkoff, H., & Loffredeo, S. (1997). *The rights of the poor: The authoritative ACLU guide to poor people's rights.* Carbondale, IL: Southern Illinois University Press.

Higgenbothem, E., & Romero, M. (Eds.) (1997). *Women and work: Exploring race, ethnicity and class: Vol. 6.* Thousand Oaks, CA: Sage.

Jencks, C. (1997). Foreword. In K. Edin & L. Lein (Eds.). *Making ends meet.* pp. ix-xxvii. New York: Russell Sage Foundation.

Jones, J. (1987). Black women, work, and the family under slavery. In N. Gerstel & H. E. Gross (Eds.), *Families and Work* (pp. 84-110). Philadelphia: Temple University Press.

Kelly, R. F., & Voyandorff, P. (1985). Work/family role strain among employed parents. *Family Relations, 34,* 367-374.

Kisker, E. E., & Ross, C. M. (1997). Arranging child care. Welfare to work. *The Future of Children, 7*(1), 99-109.

Koon, R. L. (1997). *Welfare reform. Helping the least fortunate become less dependent.* New York: Garland.

Kreuger, D. W. (1984). *Rehabilitation psychology: A comprehensive text.* Rockville, MD: Aspen.

Lamott, A. (1995). *Bird by bird: Some instructions on writing and life.* New York: Pantheon Books.

Lepak, C. R., Stokes, L., & Harder, S. (1994-1995). *Snakes and ladders: A resource manual for post-secondary students with children.* Distributed by Women in Transition and supported by an internal collaborative research project grant, University of Wisconsin-EauClaire.

Maine Equal Justice Project. (2003). Balancing the scales of justice: Welfare work and raising children. Conversations with twenty-one Maine families. Available at http://www.meip.or conversations/onestep htm

Martin-Baro I. (1994). *Writings for a liberation psychology.* In A. Aron & S. Come (Eds.). Cambridge, MA: Harvard University Press.

Masi, R., & Cooper, J. (2006). *Children's mental health: Facts for policy makers.* National Center for Children in Poverty (NCCP), Columbia University. Mailman School of Public Health. http://nccp.org/pub_ucr066.html

Miller, D. C. (1990). *Women and social welfare: A feminist analysis.* New York: Praeger.

Mink, G. (1998). *Welfare's end.* Ithaca, NY: Cornell University Press.

Mink, G., & Solinger, R. (Eds.) (2003). *Welfare: A documentary history of US policy and politics.* New York: New York University Press.

Naples, N. A. (1996). Feminist participatory research and empowerment: Going public as survivors of childhood sexual abuse. In G. Gottfried (Ed.). *Feminism and social change: Bridging theory and practice* (pp. 160-186). Chicago: University of Illinois Press.

Nathan, R. P. (1993). *Turning promises into performance: The management challenge* of *implementing Workfare.* New York: Columbia University Press.

O'Hara, B. J. (2002). Work and work-related activities of mothers receiving temporary assistance to needy families: 1996, 1998, and 2000. *Current Population Reports.* (Household Economic Studies P70-85). Washington, DC: Bureau of the CensusWashington, DC. Author.

Oliker, S. J. (1995). Work commitment and constraint among mothers on welfare. *Journal of Contemporary Ethnography, 24*(2), 165-194.

Parcel, T. L., & Menaghan, E. G. (1997). Effects of low-wage employment on family well-being. Welfare to work. *The Future of Children, 7*(1), 122-127.

Parasuraman, S., & Greenhaus, J. H. (Eds.). (1997). *Integrating work and family: Challenges and choices for a changing world.* Westport, CT: Quorum Books.

Patai, D. (1991). U. S. academics and third-world women: Is ethical research possible? In S.B. Gluck & D. Patai (Eds.).*Women's words: The feminist practice of oral history* (pp. 137-154). New York: Routledge.

Pearlin. L. (1983). Role strains and personal stress. In H. Kaplan (Ed.), *Psychosocial stress in theory and research* (pp. 3-32). New York: Academic Press.

Peck, J. (2001). *Workfare states.* New York: Guilford Press.

Perlmutter, F. D. (1997). *From welfare to work: Corporate initiatives and welfare reform.* New York: Oxford University Press.

Peterson, J. (2002 Feb.). Feminist perspectives on TANF reauthorization: An introduction to key issues for the future of welfare reform. Washington, DC: Institute for Women's Policy Research (Briefing Paper No. E511). Available at http://www.iwpr.org/pdf/e5ll.html

Polkinghorne. D. E. (1988). *Narrative knowing and the human sciences.* Albany: State University of New York Press.

Polokow, V. (1993). *Lives on the edge: Single mothers and their children in the other America.* Chicago: University of Chicago Press.

Quinn, P., & Allen, K. R. (1989). Facing challenges and making compromises: How single mothers endure. *Family Relations, 38,* 390-395.

Rank, M. (1994). *Living on the edge: The realities of welfare in America.* New York: Columbia University Press

Reik, T. (1949). *Listening with the third ear: The inner experience of a psychoanalyst.* New York: Farrar & Straus.

Rich, A. (1991). *An atlas of the difficult world: Poems, 1988-1991.* New York: W. W. Norton.

Rilke, R. M. (1985). *The sonnets of Orpheus.* (S. M. Mitchell, Trans.). New York: Simon & Schuster.

Robles, B. J. (1997). An economic profile of women in the United States. In E. Higgenbothan & M. Romero (Eds.). *Women and work: Exploring race, ethnicity, and* class: *Vol. 6* (pp. 5-27). Thousand Oaks, CA: Sage.

Roosevelt, E. (2000). *Universal declaration of human rights. Vol. 1.* Bedford, MA: Applewood Books.

Rose, N. E. (1996). *Workfare or fair work: Women. welfare. and government work programs.* Piscataway, NJ: Rutgers University Press.

Rubin, H. J., & Rubin, I. S. (1995). *Qualitative interviewing: The art of hearing data.* Thousand Oaks, CA: Sage.

Rutter, M. (1987). Psychosocial resilience and protective mechanisms. *American Journal of Orthopsychiatry, 57,* 316-331.

Schein, V. E. (1995). *Working from the margins: Voices of mothers in poverty.* Ithaca, NY: ILR Press.

Sidel, R. (1996). *Keeping women and children last.* New York: Penguin Books

Smith, S. (1995). Evaluating two-generation interventions: Current efforts and directions for future research. In S. Smith & E. Sigel (Eds.), *Two generation programs for families in poverty: A new intervention strategy. Advances in applied developmental psychology: Vol. 9* (pp. 251-270). Norwood, NJ: Ablex.

Stack, C. (1974). *All our kin.* New York: Basic Books.

Strauss, A. L. (1987). *Qualitative analysis for social scientists.* New York: Cambridge University Press.

Tedlock, B. (1995). Works and wives: On the sexual division of textual labor. In R. Behar & D.A. Gorden (Eds.), *Women writing culture* (pp. 267-286). Berkeley: University of California Press.

Turner, C. (1997). Psychosocial barriers to black women's career development. In J.V. Jordan (Ed.), *Women's growth in diversity* (pp. 162-175). New York: Guildford Press.

Turner, V. W. (1986). Dewey, Dilthey and drama: An essay in the anthropology of experience. In V. W. Turner & E. M. Bruner (Eds.). *The anthropology of experience* (pp. 33-42). Urbana, IL: University of Chicago Press.

Ury, W. (1991). *Getting past no: Negotiating your way from confrontation to cooperation.* New York: Bantam Books.

Van Manen, M. (1990). *Researching lived experience. Human science for an action sensitive pedagogy.* Albany: State University of New York Press.

Warren, J. A., & Johnson, P. J. (1995). Work-family role strain. *Family Relations, 44,* 163-169.

Watson, L. C., & Watson-Franke, M. B. (1985). *Interpreting life histories: An anthropological inquiry.* New Brunswick, NJ: Rutgers University Press.

Weil, S. (1951). *Waiting for God.* New York: Putnam.

Wittman, L., Statham, A., & Rhoades, K. (1997). *In our own words: Mothers' perspectives on welfare reform. A* project of the Women and Poverty Public Education Initiative. University of Wisconsin-Parkside.

Wittman, L. (1998). *In our own words: Mothers' needs for successful welfare reform. A* project for the Women and Poverty Public Education Initiative. Center for Community Change. University of Wisconsin-Parkside.

Wolcott, H. (1994). *Transforming qualitative data. Description analysis and interpretation.* Thousand Oaks, CA: Sage.

Zaslow, J. M., & Emig, C. A. (1997). When low-income mothers go to work: Welfare to work. *The Future of Children, 7*(1), 110-115.

doi:10.1300/J004v23n03_13

APPENDICES

Appendix A:
Cover Letter to Participants

I am a doctoral student at New York University in the Department of Occupational Therapy. As part of my requirements for my degree of Doctor of Philosophy in Occupational Therapy I am interested in studying the experiences of women who are required to participate in the mandatory Workfare program and to learn from their point of view how they are being prepared for transition to work.

The stories of women's experiences in Workfare have been rarely studied. I think it is important to hear about these experiences in order to provide information to other women who may be going through this experience and to offer direction to policy makers who can influence the program.

I am seeking to interview you about 2-3 times during the course of my study. We will schedule the interviews at your convenience.

Please read the attached consent form which will provide you with further information about the way this study will be conducted. The consent form may be returned to me by using the enclosed envelope, in person, or in the administration office.

Thank you for your time and consideration. If you have further questions, you may reach me at (212)807-0344, or if you wish you may call

[Haworth co-indexing entry note]: "Appendix A: Cover Letter to Participants." Greer, Ellen. Co-published simultaneously in *Occupational Therapy in Mental Health* (The Haworth Press, Inc.) Vol. 23, No. 3/4, 2007, pp. 181-182; and: *Women's Immersion in a Workfare Program: Emerging Challenges for Occupational Therapists* (Ellen Greer) The Haworth Press, 2007, pp. 181-182. Single or multiple copies of this article are available for a fee from The Haworth Document Delivery Service [1-800-HAWORTH, 9:00 a.m. - 5:00 p.m. (EST). E-mail address: docdelivery@haworthpress.com].

Available online at http://otmh.haworthpress.com
doi:10.1300/J004v23n03_14

Professor Deborah Labovitz, Chairperson of my dissertation committee at New York University.

Sincerely,
Ellen Greer

Appendix B:
Participant Consent Form

I have been asked by Ellen Greer to permit her to interview me about my experiences in Workfare. Ms. Greer will conduct this study as part of the requirements for the degree of Doctor of Philosophy at New York University.

I understand that my participation in this study is voluntary and that I may withdraw from the study at any time. I understand that Ms. Greer will collect data in the from of a field log and audio taped interviews.

Ms. Greer has assured me that my confidentiality will be protected: my name will not appear in any written report or publication of the study or findings. All research materials will be stored in a protected location and audio tapes will be erased at the end of the study. I understand that I retain the right to review all or any portion of an audio tape and request that it be destroyed.

I have received an unsigned copy of this form to keep and ins. Ms. Greer has answered my questions. I know that Ms. Greer will be available to answer them by reaching her at (212) 807-0344.

I also know I can contact Professor Deborah Labovitz, Ms. Greer's Chairperson at NYU at the address and phone number listed below.

Signature of Participant   Date
Signature of Investigator   Date

Deborah R Labovitz, New York University School of Education, Department of Occupational Therapy, 35 West 4th St., 11th Floor, Telephone: (212)998-5830

[Haworth co-indexing entry note]: "Appendix B: Participant Consent Form." Greer, Ellen. Co-published simultaneously in *Occupational Therapy in Mental Health* (The Haworth Press, Inc.) Vol. 23, No. 3/4, 2007, p. 183; and: *Women's Immersion in a Workfare Program: Emerging Challenges for Occupational Therapists* (Ellen Greer) The Haworth Press, 2007, p. 183. Single or multiple copies of this article are available for a fee from The Haworth Document Delivery Service [1-800-HAWORTH, 9:00 a.m. - 5:00 p.m. (EST). E-mail address: docdelivery@haworthpress.com].

Available online at http://otmh.haworthpress.com
doi:10.1300/J004v23n03_14   *183*

Appendix C:
Sample Analytic Memos and Field Log

ANALYTIC MEMOS (LOOKING AT THE DATA)

May 7, 1999
Next level of analysis–Sandra's interviews.
Went through 2nd interview and made notes in response to Sandra's narrative some general bins–looked and read through it thinking about "what are the relationships?" I ended up with an idea for a play and some realizations about Sandra in relationship with males and females–Her role as a caretaker–and wonder who is taking care of Sandra?

The next reading of both interviews will be to diagram with colored pencils, the actual stories in order–if a similar story reappears or a part of one started before I will use the same color. The purpose of this is to become clear about the stories Sandra is telling. I will then write a narrative summary of each story, then look for any themes that seem to be running through the narratives.

It has taken me a long time to figure out my method and of how I can work. I find it important to
1st reading-go through
2nd reading-line by line
3rd reading-bins
4th reading-summary or hunches or phrases that stick out-explore
5th reading-re-read with idea or theme that emerges
6th reading-make notes and react in margins-creative-significant

[Haworth co-indexing entry note]: "Appendix C: Sample Analytic Memos and Field Log." Greer, Ellen. Co-published simultaneously in *Occupational Therapy in Mental Health* (The Haworth Press, Inc.) Vol. 23, No. 3/4, 2007, pp. 185-195; and: *Women's Immersion in a Workfare Program: Emerging Challenges for Occupational Therapists* (Ellen Greer) The Haworth Press, 2007, pp. 185-195. Single or multiple copies of this article are available for a fee from The Haworth Document Delivery Service [1-800-HAWORTH, 9:00 a.m. - 5:00 p.m. (EST). E-mail address: docdelivery@haworthpress.com].

Available online at http://otmh.haworthpress.com
doi:10.1300/J004v23n03_14

7th reading–diagram narratives–write narrative summaries-pull out themes go back and re-read later–in the meantime move on to the next participant. Follow over time how this method changes, shortens.

Color coding of major narrative topics is helpful. Able to see patterns of repeating themes–Interview seems to have its own structure–formed by my opening question.

Working on a time line is going to take longer than I thought.

May 19, 1999

What stood out for me last week was within the Sandra, Pat, Ann connection. They each want out of it. I see their group function as the "mother" who cares for them in ways they didn't have. As they become strong from the care they are able to stretch out.

Ann during feeding interacted for a long time with one of the staff certified nursing assistant, she appeared to be having a serious conversation–someone Ann could look up to. She carried out the feeding activity thoughtfully until the group(her peers) wanted to leave. Ann walked away from the patient, who she was feeding with no replacement. I can imagine that she wanted to stay from the expression on her face.

Why couldn't she ask the group to wait or just say no. Ann likes being there while Sandra and Pat don't, so the group network is positive and negative-raising conflicts about fear of breaking away.

The metaphor "we keep going in a circle" comes to mind. What steps are taken to move away, what are the risks? The "circle" is status-quo safe.

June 6, 1999

Participants' Ways of Diluting the Connection to the Work Setting:

1. coming late
2. not getting the right papers
3. absence
4. falling asleep in the chair sitting with residents
5. avoiding tasks
6. isolation within one's own peer group
7. missing school because of incomplete homework
8. acting destructively on feelings of being unappreciated and injustice

Participants' Ways of Strengthening the Connection to the Work Setting:

1. coming on time
2. properly filling out the time sheets

3. getting right paper work
4. cooperating among each other
5. collaborating to get the job done
6. having lunch together
7. smoking together
8. shopping together
9. lending money when needed
10. networking for jobs
11. listening to one another
12. sharing one's life experience
13. offering perspective

I see a conflict between the "circle" and the wish to "break away."

The circle: safety

Some thoughts: the circle is the workfare process, status quo–safety, the group connection, sitting in a circle around the table, the reflective, recursive process, a symbol of unity, boundary.

Breaking Away: ambivalence

Some thoughts: from workfare, from poverty, from the group, from intimate family relationships

Participants' Ways of Coping:

Friendship
Collaboration
Getting information
Having a plan
Crying
Smoking
Eating
Exercise
Diet
Anxiety
Somatization
School

Participants' Psychological and Social Resources:

Humor
Common sense

Life experience
Ethics of care
Resilience
Ability to connect with others
To affiliate
Support networks

August, 9, 1999

Refining System of Analysis of Data

1. Read transcript notes line by line or meaning unit
2. Re-organize interview into narratives
3. Each narrative structured into stanzas
4. Re-read-on rt; side comment.
5. When completed, work backward and label left side with process
6. Write a brief summary
7. Pull out metaphors-short analysis
8. list stanzas and meaning
9. Look for pattern-major themes

ANALYTIC MEMO: REFLECTIONS

June 14, 1999

It is almost a year since I began my study at the nursing home. Reading about my entry transition, when I am now in the end stage of the project points out the integration I have experienced, as I can read the log with a cool eye, the eye of inquiry versus the eye with the pulse of emotion that also kept me from writing in a more abstract way.

What I see in this first log is an elementary structure for what will lie ahead in the year to come. In the initial binning I ask, "what is beneath the surface?" so on some level I was questioning the complexity of the workfare process, particularly in how it was playing out in the nursing home. The research opens with an introduction to Welfare by Dorothea. I become aware of the setting in the office where I get to observe a volunteer come in to report for work. I sense immediately that the time sheets are charged with intense feelings, and I do not know why, and as the year plays out, many of the conflicts are around these time sheets which prove the compliance of the volunteer so she can receive her benefit.

Camilla and Dorothea demonstrate their knowledge, perspective and way of interacting. Their separate voices come from very different places, one from privilege and the other from poverty. Their individual cultural differences are part of the what's underneath, a continual tension that the volunteers respond to, and use for separating good and bad. At the beginning of the study, Dorothea, Afro American moved from welfare status to middle class. She was the favored supervisor. She was "a hard growing girl" as many of the volunteers, and they felt understood by Dorothea. Camilla, Hispanic, and middle class was viewed by the volunteers as stigmatizing and criticizing them. By the end of the research there is a shift, which may be attributed to the fact that Dorothea takes on a more administrative role, and the volunteers no longer feel she is on their side. Instead they work together to cover each other's back.

I have noticed that when I entered the environment where I was once an insider, I struggled with feelings of being an outsider, while some of the interactions with staff have vestiges of my once insider status. Over time this completely disappears. The process of how I transition from once insider to research outsider to insider within the program is fascinating to me, as I went through many changes in my own development. Particularly from being very self-conscious about my status at the beginning to growing into the role of researcher, taking it in myself, and transforming, which over the year changed relationships, sometimes having profound consequences. I learned that change is very painful as well as joyful, and maintaining the status-quo can be much safer but stultifying.

FIELD LOG

4310 *Loç#25: April 2, 1999 (A Phone Call From Pat)*
4311 *Ellen I am calling you because some of us went to the Home Health*
4312 *Aide program and it was* horrible, *the attitude was* terrible, *and*
4313 *gave us so much stress. The teacher we had tested us every day, she read*
4314 *from a manual, and we couldn't answer the questions. The only one we*
4315 *knew was dementia, because we work with it. I tell you I was going to*
4316 *have a nervous breakdown. I almost ended up in the hospital. The way* .

4317   *she was treating us, I couldn't deal with it. She gave us a patient
       (dummy)*

4318   *in the bed, stood over us, tested us, wouldn't let us eat lunch until
       late,*

4319   *and then told me I have trouble with my back and I can't come back
       the*

4320   *next day. I can't finish the training. I had to go to the doctor, I was
       short*

4321   *of breath, my blood pressure went up, my doctor said, "what is
       wrong?*

4322   *Why are you so stressed? Whatever it is it is getting you sick.*

4323   *i would rather deal with Camilla than with this teacher, although
       Camilla*

4324   *has been rude to us. . . . The other girls had a good teacher who let
       them*

4325   *have a full stomach before they began to learn, and then she gave
       them*

4326   *time to eat lunch, and helped them learn. She didn't test them
       everyday.*

4327   *Ellen, we will all be in next Friday, please don't tell Sandra what I
       said*

4328   *because I know she wants to tell you her side of the story, and
       Ann said*

4329   *she will call you, she has been tied up with her daughter. Now we
       are*

4330   *going to take care of each other with a new plan in the day room.*

4331   *Dorothea comes up to check up on us, talks on our side, but then
       tells*

4332   *Camilla if she sees anyone not working, so now we are going to
       work in*

4333   *groups of four. Ann will work the video, and set up the movies,
       Sandra*

4334   *will work with doing exercises, I will do crafts with another group of*

4335   *residents, and Faye will talk with another group, this way we are
       always*

4336   *covered. We will take care of each other . . . I wanted you to know
       what we*

4337   are going through.

4338   *I thanked Pat for calling me, and I was glad to hear that she was
       feeling*

4339   *better and had a plan. I told her I would see her the Friday when she*

4340   *returns, to hear what happened and to go over the transcribed interviews*

4341   *for a participant check. During her conversation I had a wish to respond*

4342   *with support to what she was saying, but I have learned from the*

4343   *interviews with my participants, that when they are feeling strong*

4344   *emotions, they don't want to be stopped, my verbal reactions to what they*

4345   *are saying interferes, instead they want me to listen, and just be there. It is*

4346   *humbling. I asked a few short questions during the conversation. Pat had*

4347   *to repeat parts of her story several times until she was able to modulate*

4348   *her breath into a relaxed rhythm and finally said she was feeling better*

4349   *since she made her decision to go for further training and make the most*

4350   *of the experience before her. I need to make meaning of this*

4351   communication.

4352   Analytic Memo: April 2, 1999

4353   A few hours after writing the field log about Pat's phone call, I was

4354   thinking about her words "I just wanted you to know what we are

4355   going through" These words resonated with ideas from Simone

4356   Weil and Adrienne Rich. I go to *An Atlas of a Difficult World*, Rich's

4357   poems, 1988-1991. I find this poem:

4358   *For A Friend in Travail* (1990) pg. 51 (excerpts)

4359   *What are you going through? She said, is the great question.*

4360   *Philosopher of oppression, theorist*

4361   *Of the victories of force.*

4362   *We write from the marrow of our bones. When she did not ask, or*

4363   *tell: How victims save their own lives.*

4364   *The crawl along the ledge, then the raveling span of fibre*

4365   *Strung*

4366   *From one side to the other, I dreamed that too.*

4367   *Waking, not sure we made it. Relief, appallment, of waking.*

4368   *Consciousness. O, no. To sleep again.*

4369   *O to sleep without dreaming.*

4370   *...... What are you going through*

4371   *there on the other ledge.*

4372   *In Rich's notes she quotes Simone Weil, Waiting for God,*
        (1951)g. 115,

4373   p. 60 in Rich. "the love of our neighbor in all its fullness simply
        means

4374   being able to say to him: What are you going through?

4374   If I knew what Pat, Sandra and Ann were going through, how
        would

4375   they want me to express it in the study? With this question in
        mind, I

4376   will go over the conversation in my mind. The first image that hits
        me

4377   is the loss of trusted authorities, the bad teacher (who wouldn't let
        Pat

4378   eat lunch before her test), Camilla the supervisor who treats the

4379   volunteers rudely and takes them for granted based on the volunteers'

4379   perceptions, and Dorothea who they always counted on is now felt
        to

4380   be turning on them. All they have to survive and stay safe is each

4381   other, and within their unity is power to care and protect.

4382   The good authority (the other teacher in the training class) allows

4383   you to have a full stomach before taking on a difficult challenge, to

4384   give you needed strength. Having to do hard work while starving
        is

4385   cruelty. Was Pat telling me how hard life is for them overall with
        the

4386   food insecurity issues among the many obstacles they face daily,
        and

4387   her need to be fed emotionally by a kind and beneficent authority?

4388   Maybe the others will tell me they're perspective of the training

4389   experience on Friday.

4391   *Los# 29 June 4, 1999*

4392   Today was my third visit since Log #28.1 made notes-handwrit-
        ten.

4393   Essentially I went back to the nursing home to fill in the gaps, to do
        a

4394   participant check, and to get a better sense of the program. I feel I
        have

4395   taken the micro view for a year and now I need to shift perspective.

4395   My notes focused on the daily schedule of volunteer activities in the
        day

4396 room on the half hour. This gives the day structure and defines the
4397 volunteers' responsibilities. At lunch time, the volunteers go out to buy
4398 lunch and then return and eat together at a long table in the cafeteria.
4399 There are other tables as well and volunteers sit in cliques, new volunteers
4400 sit separately form the more experienced volunteers. There is an
4401 unspoken hierarchy based on duration of time at the work site. The older
4402 volunteers won't have anything to do with the new ones.
4403 At the lunch table, talk is about giving birth, children, sons in jail, and
4404 criticizing Camillas' parenting of her son. Sometimes a package of
4405 cookies is offered to someone. Ann brings her lunch always concerned
4406 with cholesterol, Pat eats turkey because she has high blood pressure and
4407 has to watch her weight, and Sandra will eat Kentucky Fried Chicken.
4408 Sandra is now in the Pep program, and didn't come today because she
4409 didn't get her transportation money. Ann and Pat were in today, and I
4410 joined them at the end of their lunch. The lunchroom was empty, they
4411 were sitting at the table with a relatively new volunteer Mona. Pat was
4412 talking about her experience when she had her first abortion, and how she
4413 had a breakdown, how her mother observed what she went through and
4414 treated her like a princess for the second pregnancy. The women talked
4415 about their feelings about mothers, pregnancy and abortion.
4416 Mona said the problem is that girls can't talk to their mothers, they are
4417 afraid to talk to their mothers about being pregnant, remember Tara, her
4418 mother beat her, hit her in her stomach, she beat that girl, and she ran

4419   away, her friend told her, get out of there, don't stand for that abuse.

4420   Mona went on, that when she told her mother she was pregnant, her

4421   mother was wonderful. She said, "I always tell my mother everything, I

4422   always go to her for advice, when I first told her I could see that she was

4423   going to cry, but she supported me and told me I had to go on welfare.

4424   Ann said, "I didn't want to go on welfare, I was working but my mother

4425   took me down, and got me on. Abortion doesn't bother me, as long as you

4426   have them before three months I had five, I would never have an abortion

4427   after three months, I couldn't do it." Mona was saying that she doesn't

4428   want to have any more children, not if she is on public assistance.

4429   This conversation continued later on in the day room during the movie

4430   hour. Ann was saying, "It embarrasses me when I tell people I've been

4431   here for two years and I haven't been hired. This August single people are

4432   getting taken off, all they'll get is help with rent, no cash. I don't know

4433   what I'll do without cash, I have to get a job . . . . . .

4434   Another topic that came up is how they are going to find a job. This

4435   summer both Pat and Ann are sending their children away, and are

4436   considering doing this permanently, given he uncertainty of their

4437   situation once the benefit is up. So they are thinking ahead how they are

4438   going to manage, and they realize they won't be able to provide for their

4439   children. Ann reported: I am going to work at the amusement park this

4440 summer with Sandra. I stay at Sandra's house or my sisters. I'll get

4441 revenge on my older kids, I'm shutting the cable, no food in the

4442 refrigerator, and I'll have my large travel bag with everything in it so I can

4443 stay in Brooklyn. I went for the interview and spoke with a nice white

4444 man. Then I visited Sandra, had some soup, and met her nephew.

doi:10.1300/J004v23n03_14

Index

T - #0242 - 101024 - C0 - 212/152/12 [14] - CB - 9780789030283 - Gloss Lamination